"A MUST HAVE GUIDE"

HEALTH DOCTOR

THE SECRET TO A HEALTHY LIFESTYLE

UNIVERSAL LEARNING ACADEMY

DEDICATION

THIS BOOK IS DEDICATED TO **YOU** THE READER TO HELP
YOU TO LIVE A HEALTHIER LIFESTYLE!

First Published in UK in 2016
Published by DVG STAR Publishing

www.UniversalLearningAcademy.com

Disclaimer

CONTENTS

ACKNOWLEDGMENTS

Our sincere appreciation to the Universal Learning Academy team for collating this very useful book on the benefits of fruits, vegetables, spices and herbs. Thank you to DVG STAR Publishers for publishing this book.

FRUITS

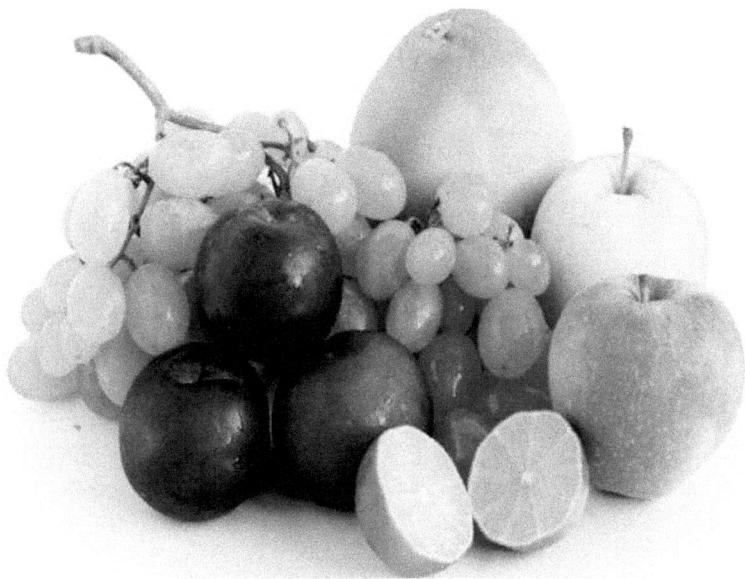

UNIVERSAL LEARNING ACADEMY

HEALTH BENEFITS OF FRUITS

Fruits are nature's wonderful gifts. These have a lot of vitamins and minerals, fibre and different phytochemicals. They are low in calories and fat. Think about these delicious colourful fruits: red, green, orange and yellow.

These differently coloured fruits have different phytochemicals which act as antioxidants that help to eliminate free radicals from the body. Free radicals are the main causative molecules that induce cancer causing cell proliferation. These free radicals form during metabolic activities in the cells due to environmental exposure to tobacco smoke, radiation, and some chemicals like mercury. These free radicals have the ability to damage the DNA in the cells and the protein in the cell membrane. This effect may cause the development of cancer cells in the damaged area.

Researchers have found that the phytochemicals in fruits, vegetables and spices act as antioxidants and detoxify these free radicals. Therefore if we eat these colourful fruits they will reduce the risk of diseases like cancer, heart disease, eye disease (cataract), and age related macular degeneration. They also reduce the effect of Alzheimer's disease, and delay aging and wrinkling of the skin.

The latest research has suggested that an element known as selenium is essential for the formation of an antioxidant enzyme that detoxifies free radicals.

Some fruits naturally contain selenium. Fruits act as natural vitamin tonics; if you eat at least one green, orange, yellow or red fruit and vegetables per day (that is, eat seven types a day) you can keep the doctor away and live a long and healthy life.

What are these colours? These colours are due to phytochemicals which act as powerful antioxidants in the human body.

Red fruits contain lycopene and anthocyanin, which are powerful antioxidant phytochemicals.

(These are in red grapes, red apples, and strawberries)

Orange and Yellow fruits contain lutein, zeaxanthin and carotenoids.

(In bananas, papaya, mangoes, oranges, lemons and, pineapples)

Green fruits contain phytochemicals like saponin and indole.

(In green grapes, avocados and green apples)

Purple/Blue fruits contain anthocyanin.

(In apples, grapes, and berries)

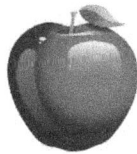

APPLE

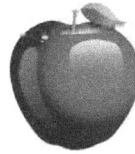

NUTRITION FACTS

VITAMINS – Vitamin C (4.6mg), Thiamin (0.017mg), Riboflavin (0.026mg), Niacin (0.091mg), Vitamins B6 (0.041mg), Folate (3μg), Vitamin A (3μg), Vitamin E (0.18mg) and Vitamin K (2.2μg).

MINERALS – Calcium (6mg), Iron (0.12mg), Magnesium (5mg), Phosphorus (11mg), Potassium (107mg), Sodium (1 mg) and Zinc (0.04mg).

[USDA national nutrient database, 2015]

Nutrient	Value per 100g
Energy	52kcal
Protein	0.26g
Fat	0.17g
Carbohydrate	13.81g
Fibre	2.4g
Sugar	10.39g

HEALTH BENEFITS

☆ **Antioxidant benefits**

☆ **Cardiovascular benefits**

☆ **Relief from constipation**

☆ **Prevent tooth decay**

☆ **Protects the brain from damage**

☆ **Helps to reduce mental stress**

☆ **Blood sugar regulation**

☆ **Anti-cancer**

☆ **Anti-inflammatory benefits**

☆ **May decrease risk of type 2 diabetes**

☆ **Regulates immune response**

☆ **Helps weight loss**

☆ **Anti-asthma**

Apples are rich in vitamins, minerals and antioxidants, which are essential for a healthy life.

Apples contain soluble fibre called pectin which lowers high cholesterol levels in blood, helps in easy digestion and gives relief from constipation.

Acids in apples exert an antiseptic germ present in the mouth and prevent tooth decay.

Vitamin C in apples is a powerful antioxidant; it protects the brain from damage. The antioxidant in apples is called quercetin; it reduces the effect of free radicals and protects the brain cells, thus reducing mental stress.

Antioxidant benefits of apples are that they decrease oxidation of cell membrane fats. This benefit is especially important in our cardiovascular system since oxidation of fat (called lipid peroxidation) in the membranes of cells that line our blood vessels is a primary risk factor for clogging of the arteries (atherosclerosis) and other cardiovascular problems. Apples' strong antioxidant benefits are also related to their ability to lower risk of asthma in numerous studies, and their ability to lower risk of lung cancer.

Apples contain phytochemicals including quercetin, catechin, phloridzin, and chlorogenic acid, all of which are strong antioxidants. These phytochemicals may inhibit cancer cell proliferation, and regulate inflammatory and immune response.

Apples can help prevent various diseases such as cancer, heart disease, asthma, diabetes, and weight loss.

Cardiovascular benefits are associated with two aspects of apple nutrients: their water-soluble fibre (pectin) content, and their unusual mix of polyphenols. Decreased lipid peroxidation is a key factor in lowering risk of many chronic heart problems.

Cardiovascular disease and cancer are thought to be the results of oxidative stress. Apples are a good source of antioxidants. These antioxidants help to prevent oxidative stress and may therefore help prevent these chronic diseases. Apples contain quercetin, a powerful antioxidant which is associated with reducing the risk.

It was found that catechin, another flavonoid found in apples, is also associated with decreased epithelial lung cancer.

Flavonoids provide a 35% reduction in the risk of cardiovascular diseases and reduced risk of death from coronary heart disease.

Anti-cancer benefits is also a key factor of apples. Apples have shown to help colon and breast cancer but the most prominent one is lung cancer.

Blood sugar regulation is benefited by having an apple a day. The polyphenols found in apples are capable of influencing our digestion and absorption of carbohydrates, and the overall impact of these changes is to improve regulation of our blood sugar. The impact of apple polyphenols on our body include:

- Slowing down of carbohydrate digestion. Carbohydrates are broken down less readily into simple sugars, and less load is placed on our bloodstream to accommodate more sugar.

- Reduction of glucose absorption.

- Stimulation of the pancreas to put out more insulin.

- Stimulation of insulin receptors to latch on to more insulin and increase the flow of sugar out of our bloodstream and into our cells.

Anti-asthma benefits of apples are definitely associated with the antioxidant and anti-inflammatory nutrients found in this fruit.

Apple intake reduces the risk of asthma and decreases bronchial hyper sensitivity, therefore increasing lung function.

Other health benefits include macular degeneration of the eye and neurodegenerative problems, including Alzheimer's disease. Higher quercetin levels may decrease the risk of type 2 diabetes, and the quercetin found in apples is considered to be associated with weight loss in overweight women.

BANANA

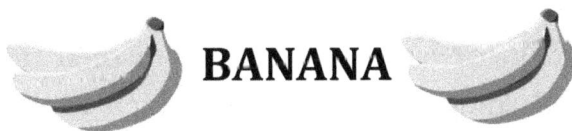

NUTRITION FACTS

VITAMINS – Vitamin C (8.7mg),
Thiamin (0.031mg), Riboflavin (0.073mg),
Niacin (0.665mg), Vitamin B6 (0.367mg),
Folate (20µg), Vitamin A (3µg),
Vitamin E (0.1mg) and Vitamin K (0.5µg).

MINERALS – Calcium (5mg),
Iron (0.26mg), Magnesium (27mg),
Phosphorus (22mg), Potassium (358mg),
Sodium (1 mg) and Zinc (0.15mg).

[USDA national nutrient database, 2015]

Nutrient	Value per 100g
Energy	89kcal
Protein	1.09g
Fat	0.33g
Carbohydrate	22.84g
Fibre	2.6g
Sugar	12.23g

HEALTH BENEFITS

☆ **Cardiovascular benefits**

☆ **Helps prevent high blood pressure**

☆ **Protects against atherosclerosis**

☆ **Strengthens teeth and bones**

☆ **Helps reduce anaemia**

☆ **Digestive benefits**

☆ **Boosts energy**

☆ **Relief from constipation**

☆ **Helps prevent night blindness**

Bananas are a good source of both vitamins and minerals, as well as fibre.

Cardiovascular benefit of bananas is related to their potassium content. Bananas are a good source of potassium, which is an essential mineral for maintaining normal blood pressure and heart function. Having a banana a day will help to prevent high blood pressure and protect against atherosclerosis.

Sterol content, a type of fat found in small quantities in bananas also plays an important role in preventing cardiovascular diseases. Sterol look structurally similar to cholesterol and can block the absorption of dietary cholesterol. By blocking absorption, they help us maintain our blood cholesterol at a healthy level.

The amount of fibre content found in bananas is another contributing factor to a healthy cardiovascular system. Soluble fibre in food is associated with decreased risk of heart disease, thus regular intake of bananas are potentially helpful in lowering the risks of getting any heart diseases.

Digestive benefits of bananas is that they have a low glycemic index (GI) value. GI measures the impact of a food on our blood sugar. This low GI value for bananas is most likely related to two of their carbohydrate-related qualities.

The amount of fibre found in bananas help regulate the speed of digestion, and by keeping digestion well-regulated, conversion of carbohydrates to simple sugars and release of simple sugars from digesting foods also stays well-regulated.

Within their total fibre content, bananas also contain pectins. Pectins are unique and complicated types of fibre. Some of the components in pectins are water-soluble, and others are not. As bananas ripen, their water-soluble pectins increase, and this helps normalize the rate of carbohydrate digestion and moderates the impact of banana consumption on our blood sugar.

The soluble fibre content in bananas not only helps digestion it also provides relief from constipation.

Bananas have a high amount of potassium which is a component of body fluid and helps in maintaining heart rate and blood pressure by counteracting the bad effects of sodium. Bananas contain vitamin B6 and folate which are essential for the formation of red blood cells and help reduce anaemia. Vitamin K is essential for the clotting of blood. Calcium and phosphorous, on the other hand, help in strengthening bones and teeth.

Tryptophan is an amino acid found in bananas, which is converted to serotonin by our body. Serotonin helps in relaxing the mind, the brain, and the nervous system, and also regulates the mood, thus reducing tension of the body and mind, making one feel happy.

Thus phytochemicals such as lutein-zeaxanthin, alpha-carotene act as antioxidants and reduce the bad effects of free radicals and protect the body. Carotene is essential for good vision and reduces the risk of night blindness.

Bananas are concentrated with easily digestible simple sugars that give instant energy. This fruit is most popular amongst athletes due to its unique mix of vitamins, minerals, and low glycemic carbohydrates.

"AN APPLE A DAY KEEPS THE DOCTOR AWAY"

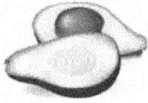

AVOCADO

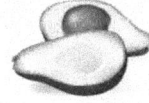

NUTRITION FACTS

VITAMINS – Vitamin C (10mg), Thiamin (0.067mg), Riboflavin (0.13mg), Niacin (1.738mg), Vitamin B6 (0.257mg), Folate (81µg), Vitamin A (7µg), Vitamin E (2.07mg) and Vitamin K (21µg).

MINERALS – Calcium (12mg), Iron (0.55mg), Magnesium (29mg), Phosphorus (52mg), Potassium (485mg), Sodium (7mg) and Zinc (0.64mg).

[USDA national nutrient database, 2015]

Nutrient	Value per 100g
Energy	160kcal
Protein	2g
Fat	14.66g
Carbohydrate	8.53g
Fibre	6.7g
Sugar	0.66g

HEALTH BENEFITS

☆ **Eases arthritis symptoms and osteoarthritis related pain**

☆ **Reduces risk of certain cancers**

☆ **Lowers cholesterol**

☆ **Boosts eye health**

☆ **Cardiovascular benefits**

☆ **Anti-inflammatory benefits**

☆ **Beneficial for pregnant women**

☆ **Helps prevent constipation**

Even though avocados have a high fat content, it's a great source of potassium, omega-3 fatty acids and lutein. It also comprises of good amounts of soluble and insoluble fibres. Consumption of an avocado helps prevent constipation.

Avocados consist of phytosterols, carotenoid antioxidants, omega 3 fatty acids, and polyhydroxolated fatty alcohols, which make the fruit an anti-inflammatory agent. Avocados are believed to help with arthritis and osteoarthritis-related pains.

Consumption of avocados helps reduce the risk of certain cancers, such as mouth, skin and prostate, as it possess a mix of antioxidant and anti-inflammatory characteristics. Avocados contain rich sources of both vitamin E and glutathione which is beneficial during chemotherapy because chemotherapy tends to reduce glutathione storage supply and thus avocados are a great way to get that antioxidant back into the system.

Avocados are also beneficial in lowering blood cholesterol levels as it contains high levels of beta-sitosterol, monounsaturated fat, which is a compound that lowers blood cholesterol levels.

Avocados contain phytonutrients such as lutein, and zeaxanthin that are essential for healthy eyes. Lutein and zeaxanthin are carotenoids, that act as antioxidants in the eye, lowering risk of developing age-related eye conditions. Thus daily consumption of avocados can protect the tissues of the eye from sun damage and the formation of cataracts and macular degeneration. It is the fat content in avocado that helps the body absorb the carotenoid.

The high content of vitamin B6 and folic acid in avocados help to reduce blood cholesterol levels thus reducing the overall risk for heart disease as well as to help prevent birth defects.

The rich fibre content of the avocado will help you feel full faster and for a longer period of time, making it a weight loss aid.

The benefits of this naturally nutrient-dense fruit will help you stay healthy and live longer.

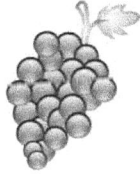

GRAPES

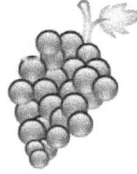

NUTRITION FACTS

VITAMINS – Vitamin C (3.2mg), Thiamin (0.069mg), Riboflavin (0.07mg), Niacin (0.188mg), Vitamin B6 (0.086mg), Folate (2μg), Vitamin A (3μg), Vitamin E (0.19mg) and Vitamin K (14.6μg).

MINERALS – Calcium (10mg), Iron (0.36mg), Magnesium (7mg), Phosphorus (20mg), Potassium (191mg), Sodium (2mg) and Zinc (0.07mg).

[USDA national nutrient database, 2015]

Nutrient	Value per 100g
Energy	69kcal
Protein	0.72g
Fat	0.16g
Carbohydrate	18.1g
Fibre	0.9g
Sugar	15.48g

HEALTH BENEFITS

☆ **Antioxidant benefits**

☆ **Anti-inflammatory benefits**

☆ **Helps reduce risk of heart attacks**

☆ **Reduces blood clots**

☆ **Can help cure migraines**

☆ **Eliminates toxins from the body**

☆ **Helps boost body's immune system**

☆ **Reduces kidney stress**

☆ **Reduces tumour cells**

☆ **Reduces constipation**

☆ **Anti-aging and longevity benefits**

☆ **Cognitive benefits**

☆ **Anti-microbial benefits**

☆ **Anti-cancer benefits**

Grapes have lots of vitamins, minerals and powerful antioxidant phytochemicals.

The fibre and organic acids in grapes reduce constipation and clean the digestive system.

Resveratrol, a phytochemical in grapes, increases the nitric oxide level in blood that prevents blood clots and causes relaxation in blood vessels, thus reducing the risk of heart attacks.

The iron content of the body is increased by regular consumption of grapes, which also reduces the anaemic condition of the body. The antioxidants in grapes help to boost the body's immune system.

Grapes help to eliminate uric acid in urine and reduce kidney stress.

Saponin present in the skin of green grapes prevents the absorption of cholesterol and reduces blood cholesterol levels.

Resveratrol is a powerful antioxidant that reduces breast cancer. It has been discovered in laboratory specimens that resveratrol reduces tumour cells. It also reduces prostate cancer by inhibiting the growth of tumour cells. Resveratrol helps to regenerate brain cells.

Grape juice helps to prevent age related macular degeneration in eyes and loss of vision.

Anthocyanin, a powerful antioxidant in grapes, has anti-allergic, anti-inflammatory, anti-microbial, and anti-cancer activity. Anthocyanin inhibits the growth of cancer cells.

It has been found that grape juice can cure migraines. It should be consumed early in the morning without mixing with water.

Grapes are very effective at eliminating toxins from the body and cleansing the blood.

"TAKE CARE OF YOUR BODY AND IT WILL TAKE CARE OF YOU"

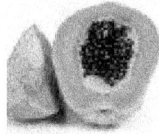

PAPAYA

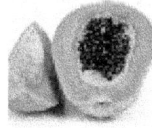

NUTRITION FACTS

VITAMINS – Vitamin C (60.9mg), Thiamin (0.023mg), Riboflavin (0.027mg), Niacin (0.357mg), Vitamin B6 (0.038mg), Folate (37µg), Vitamin A (47µg), Vitamin E (0.3mg) and Vitamin K (2.6µg).

MINERALS – Calcium (20mg), Iron (0.25mg), Magnesium (21mg), Phosphorus (10mg), Potassium (182mg), Sodium (8mg) and Zinc (0.08mg).

[USDA national nutrient database, 2015]

Nutrient	Value per 100g
Energy	43kcal
Protein	0.47g
Fat	0.26g
Carbohydrate	10.82g
Fibre	1.7g
Sugar	7.82g

HEALTH BENEFITS

☆ Protection against heart disease

☆ Protects against risk of certain cancers

☆ Anti-asthma

☆ Helps prevent diabetes

☆ Helps maintain a healthy heart rate and blood pressure

☆ Promotes digestive health and prevents constipation

☆ Anti-inflammatory effects

☆ Immune support

☆ Protection against macular degeneration

☆ Protection against rheumatoid arthritis

☆ **Healthy skin, hair and vision**

☆ **Heals wounds**

Papaya has vitamins A, B, C, E and K. They act as a tonic and rejuvenate the body.

Papaya has soluble fibre that helps easy bowel movement and reduces constipation. Papain enzyme in this fruit promotes the digestion of protein. In traditional medicine this ripe fruit was used to cure all kinds of stomach ailments and to reduce inflammation of the liver and spleen.

Potassium in this fruit is an important component of body fluid and helps in maintaining heart rate and blood pressure. Vitamin A in papaya is essential for healthy skin, mucous membranes and vision.

Beta-carotene and vitamin C are powerful antioxidants which help to reduce free radicals in the body and protect the body from the risk of cardiovascular diseases, as well as oral, prostate and lung cancer.

It has been found that vitamin A is essential for the visual cycle, reproduction, epithelial function, growth and development. Lutein is an antioxidant that protects the body from colon cancer, prostate cancer, and breast cancer. Beta-carotene in papaya prevents the symptoms of aging and wrinkling of the skin and helps in maintaining glowing skin.

Antioxidant, zeaxanthin, found in papaya, filters out harmful blue light rays and is thought to play a protective role in eye health and prevent damage from macular degeneration.

The risks for developing asthma are lowered in people who consume a high amount of certain nutrients such as beta-carotene, found in foods like papaya, apricots, broccoli and carrots.

Fibre content in papayas help prevent diabetes. Certain studies have shown that people with type 1 diabetes who consume high fibre diets have lower blood glucose levels and people with type 2 diabetes may have improved blood sugar, lipids and insulin levels.

Chronic inflammation is reduced by having a papaya as it contains a very important and versatile nutrient known as choline. Choline also aids our bodies in sleep, muscle movement, learning, memory, helps to maintain the structure of cellular membranes, aids in the transmission of nerve impulses and assists in the absorption of fat.

Research has shown that proteolytic enzymes chymopapain and papain found in papaya appears to be beneficial for promoting wound healing and preventing infection of burned areas when used topically.

Vitamin A present in papaya is great for your hair as it's a nutrient required for sebum production that keeps hair moisturized. Vitamin A is also necessary for the growth of all bodily tissues, including skin and hair.

Adequate intake of vitamin C, present in papaya, is required to help build and maintain collagen, which provides structure to skin and hair.

"YOU ARE WHAT YOU EAT FROM YOUR HEAD DOWN TO YOUR FEET"

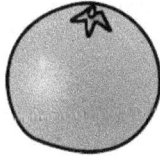

ORANGE

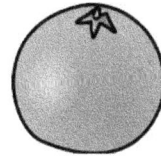

NUTRITION FACTS

VITAMINS – Vitamin C (53.2mg), Thiamin (0.087mg), Riboflavin (0.04mg), Niacin (0.282mg), Vitamin B6 (0.06mg), Folate (30μg), Vitamin A (11μg) and Vitamin E (0.18mg)

MINERALS – Calcium (40mg), Iron (0.1mg), Magnesium (10mg), Phosphorus (14mg), Potassium (181mg), and Zinc (0.07mg).

[USDA national nutrient database, 2015]

Nutrient	Value per 100g
Energy	47kcal
Protein	0.94g
Fat	0.12g
Carbohydrate	11.75g
Fibre	2.4g
Sugar	9.35g

HEALTH BENEFITS

☆ **Antioxidant benefits**

☆ **Immune support**

☆ **Cardiovascular benefits**

☆ **Lower cholesterol**

☆ **Easy digestion and reduces constipation**

☆ **Acts as a tonic and cure for fever**

☆ **Protects the kidneys**

☆ **Help prevent ulcers**

☆ **Helps maintain a healthy blood pressure**

☆ **Prevents symptoms of aging**

☆ **Healthier bones and teeth**

☆ **Anti-cancer**

☆ **Protection against rheumatoid arthritis**

Oranges are a citrus fruit, rich in vitamin C. Vitamin C is a powerful antioxidant that boosts the immune system of our body and induces disease resistance ability. High concentrations of vitamin C protect our body cells from the damage caused by free radicals. Orange juice induces the secretion of digestive juices in the colon, and helps in easy digestion and bowel movements, reducing constipation.

The pectin fibre in oranges is a laxative and protects the mucus membrane of the colon by decreasing the exposure to toxic metabolic products in the colon. The carbohydrates in oranges are fruit sugars that are easily digestible and give energy within half an hour. Orange juice, therefore, is a good kind of fruit juice for many types of fever. It has minerals which act as a tonic and cure fever.

Iron, folate and vitamin B6 are essential for the synthesis of haemoglobin and red blood cells in the blood. Haemoglobin is essential for carrying oxygen in the blood.

'Hesperidin' in the orange is a flavonoid type of phytochemical that reduces cholesterol levels in the blood and regulates blood pressure. High concentrations of vitamin C also maintain blood pressure.

Potassium in the orange is a component of body fluid. It helps in counteracting the sodium level in blood and maintains blood pressure.

Beta-carotene a powerful antioxidant in oranges which protects the skin cells from getting damaged by free radicals, thus it prevents the symptoms of aging and wrinkling. It helps in maintaining shiny skin.

Liminoid, a phytochemical in oranges and the high concentration of vitamin C in oranges reduce the activity of free radicals and prevent cancer in the mouth, colon, skin, lungs, and breast.

Orange juice induces urinary output and reduces the risk of calcium oxalate stone formation in the kidneys; orange juice thus protects the kidneys.

Calcium and phosphorus in oranges keep bones and teeth healthy. Vitamin A is good for vision and reduces the risk of night blindness. Vitamin A, C, lutein, hesperidin and liminoid are powerful antioxidants that remove the free radicals' activity in the cells and protect our body.

"STOP SAYING I WISH, START SAYING I WILL"

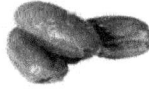

DATES

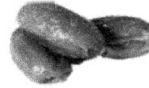

NUTRITION FACTS

VITAMINS – Thiamin (0.05mg), Riboflavin (0.06mg), Niacin (1.61mg), Vitamin B6 (0.249mg), Folate (15μg), Vitamin A (7μg) and Vitamin K (2.7μg).

MINERALS – Calcium (64mg), Iron (0.9mg), Magnesium (54mg), Phosphorus (62mg), Potassium (696mg), Sodium (1mg) and Zinc (0.44mg).

[USDA national nutrient database, 2015]

Nutrient	Value per 100g
Energy	277kcal
Protein	1.81g
Fat	0.15g
Carbohydrate	74.97g
Fibre	6.7g
Sugar	66.47g

HEALTH BENEFITS

☆ **Promoting digestive health and relief from constipation**

☆ **Cardiovascular benefits**

☆ **Anti-inflammatory benefits**

☆ **Helps reduce blood pressure**

☆ **Helps reduce the risk of strokes**

☆ **Helps to provide a healthy pregnancy and delivery**

☆ **Boosts brain health**

Dates are great for weight loss, relieving constipation, supporting regular bowel movements, promoting heart health, reducing heart disease risk, diarrhea, iron-deficiency anemia, reducing blood pressure, impotence, promoting respiratory and digestive health, pregnancy deliveries, hemorrhoid prevention, chronic conditions such as arthritis, reducing colitis risk and preventing colon cancer.

Dates contain essential nutrients, vitamins, minerals, and antioxidants for healthy growth.

Dates are a good source of iron, which is essential for the synthesis of haemoglobin.

Haemoglobin in red blood cells carries oxygen all over the body. Dates are a good source of potassium, which is a component of body fluid that controls heart rate and blood pressure. The fibre in dates prevents low density cholesterol (LDL) absorption in the gut and prevents heart disease. It contains easily digestible sugars; when eaten they release energy and give strength immediately.

Vitamin A in dates is good for vision and essential for healthy mucous membranes and skin.

Calcium in dates is necessary for healthy bones and teeth, muscular function, and nerve conduction.

Tannin in dates has anti-infective and anti-inflammatory properties, and increases the immunity of the body. Beta-carotene and lutein are antioxidants that protect the cells in the body from free radicals.

Zeaxanthin in dates is good for the retina and protects the eyes from age related macular degeneration. Lutein protects the body from colon cancer, prostate cancer, breast cancer and pancreatic cancer.

Dates have many vitamins and minerals and work as a tonic for all age groups.

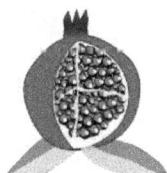

POMEGRANATE

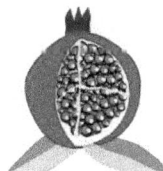

NUTRITION FACTS

VITAMINS – Vitamin C (10.2mg), Thiamin (0.067mg), Riboflavin (0.053mg), Niacin (0.293mg), Vitamin B6 (0.075mg), Folate (38µg), Vitamin E (0.6mg) and Vitamin K (16.4µg)

MINERALS – Calcium (10mg), Iron (0.3mg), Magnesium (12mg), Phosphorus (36mg), Potassium (236mg), Sodium (3mg) and Zinc (0.35mg).

[USDA national nutrient database, 2015]

Nutrient	Value per 100g
Energy	83kcal
Protein	1.67g
Fat	1.17g
Carbohydrate	18.7g
Fibre	4g
Sugar	13.67g

HEALTH BENEFITS

☆ **Prevents heart disease**

☆ **Lowers blood pressure**

☆ **May help prevent cancer**

☆ **Help digestion**

☆ **Boosts immunity**

☆ **Anti-aging**

☆ **Lowers stress levels**

☆ **Keep Alzheimer's at bay**

☆ **Prevents plaque formation**

This fruit is a good source of vitamin B complex, is a high source of other vitamins and minerals, and is considered a medicinal fruit. This fruit contains a large quantity of soluble and insoluble fibre, which helps in easy digestion and reduces constipation.

Pomegranates are a good source of vitamin C, a powerful antioxidant which helps the body develop resistance against infectious factors and inhibits viral infection.

Pomegranate juice contains ellagitannin, a tannin type of poly phenolic compound which is a powerful antioxidant. This removes free radicals from the cells and reduces heart disease risk factors. This juice reduces systolic blood pressure by inhibiting particular enzyme activity and reduces bad cholesterol levels in the blood.

Regular intake of pomegranate juice has been found to be effective against prostate cancer and diabetes, and ellagitannin can slow down the progression of cancer cells.

Pomegranate juice with honey is good for memory and the regeneration of brain cells. Anthocyanin, another phytochemical in this juice, is a powerful antioxidant, having an anti-bacterial effect and removes free radicals from the cells. The soluble fibre delays glucose absorption in the small intestine and helps to control diabetes.

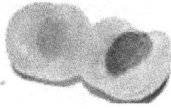

APRICOT

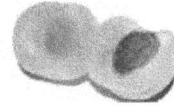

NUTRITION FACTS

VITAMINS – Vitamin C (10mg), Thiamin (0.03mg), Riboflavin (0.04mg), Niacin (0.6mg), Vitamin B6 (0.054mg), Folate (9µg), Vitamin A (96µg), Vitamin E (0.89mg) and Vitamin K (3.3µg)

MINERALS – Calcium (13mg), Iron (0.39mg), Magnesium (10mg), Phosphorus (23mg), Potassium (259mg), Sodium (1mg) and Zinc (0.2mg).

[USDA national nutrient database, 2015]

Nutrient	Value per 100g
Energy	48kcal
Protein	1.4g
Fat	0.39g
Carbohydrate	11.12g
Fibre	2g
Sugar	9.24g

HEALTH BENEFITS

☆ **Antioxidant benefits**

☆ **Protects eyesight**

☆ **Anti-inflammatory benefits**

☆ **Rich source of antioxidants**

☆ **Healthy digestive tract**

☆ **Cardiovascular benefits**

☆ **Control cholesterol levels**

☆ **Controls blood pressure**

Apricots are rich in many plant antioxidants. that provides you with the protective effects while adding very few calories to your daily total.

Apricots are rich in other antioxidants too, including polyphenolic antioxidants like flavonoids. These have been linked to a reduction in heart diseases.

Research has shown that apricots are also rich in carotenoids and xanthophylls, nutrients that have been believed to help protect eyesight from aging-related damage

Apricots are a good source of both vitamin A (from beta-carotene) and vitamin C.

Apricots are a strong dietary source of catechins, a broad family of flavonoid phytonutrients which are known to be potent anti-inflammatory. Research has shown that these nutrients inhibit the activity of an enzyme called cyclooxygenase-2 (COX-2), one of the critical steps in the process of inflammation.

High levels of catechins means that the consumption of apricots can protect blood vessels from inflammation-related damage, leading to better blood pressure control.

Other health benefits are from the rich source of fibre content which supports a healthy digestive tract and help control cholesterol levels.

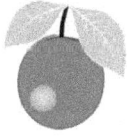

BLUEBERRIES

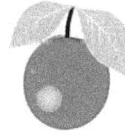

NUTRITION FACTS

VITAMINS – Vitamin C (9.7mg),
Thiamin (0.037mg), Riboflavin (0.041mg),
Niacin (0.418mg), Vitamin B6 (0.052mg),
Folate (6µg), Vitamin A (3µg),
Vitamin E (0.57mg) and Vitamin K (19.3µg)

MINERALS – Calcium (6mg),
Iron (0.28mg), Magnesium (6mg),
Phosphorus (12mg), Potassium (77mg),
Sodium (1mg) and Zinc (0.16mg).

[USDA national nutrient database, 2015]

Nutrient	Value per 100g
Energy	57kcal
Protein	0.74g
Fat	0.33g
Carbohydrate	14.49g
Fibre	2.4g
Sugar	9.96g

HEALTH BENEFITS

- ☆ **Antioxidant benefits**
- ☆ **Maintaining healthy bones**
- ☆ **Helps lower blood pressure**
- ☆ **Managing diabetes**
- ☆ **Helps prevent heart diseases**
- ☆ **Prevents constipation and promotes a healthy digestive tract**
- ☆ **Anti-aging**
- ☆ **Anti-cancer**

The most important health benefit found in blueberries involves their phytonutrient content. Anthocyanins (the colourful antioxidant pigments that give many foods their wonderful shades of blue, purple, and red) are usually the first phytonutrients to be mentioned in descriptions of blueberries and their amazing health-supportive properties. The phytonutrients function both as antioxidants and as anti-inflammatory compounds in the body, and they are responsible for many of the health benefits associated with blueberries.

Research has shown that the consumption of blueberries improved antioxidant defences in body systems that need special protection from oxidative stress, like the cardiovascular system. The most important aspect is not only the cardiovascular system that has been shown to have strengthened antioxidant status following consumption of blueberries but its's virtually every body system. For example, there is new evidence that damage to muscles following heavy exercise can be reduced through consumption of blueberries.

The nervous system can also benefit from regular consumption of blueberries. It's this whole body antioxidant support that helps blueberries stand out as an amazing antioxidant fruit.

Research studies have shown that blueberries help to improve blood fat balances, including reduction in total cholesterol, raising of high density lipoproteins (HDL) cholesterol, and lowering of triglycerides. As well as helping to protect the blood components (like LDL cholesterol) from oxygen damage that could lead to eventual clogging of the blood vessels. Protection has also been shown for the cells lining the blood vessel walls.

Regular blueberry intake has been shown to support healthy blood pressure. In individuals with high blood pressure, blueberry intake has significantly reduced both systolic and diastolic blood pressures. In individuals with health blood pressure, blueberry intake has been shown to help maintain these healthy pressures.

By lowering the risk of oxidative stress in our nerve cells, blueberries also help us maintain smoothly working nerve cells thus resulting in a healthy cognitive function.

Consumption of blueberries have shown to have a favourable impact on blood sugar regulation in individuals who have already been diagnosed with diabetes.

The retina of the eye is a unique place in our body and it is also a place that is at higher than normal risk of oxidative stress. Daily consumption of blueberries also help the retina from oxygen damage.

Anti-cancer benefits have also been distinguished with blueberries such as breast cancer, colon cancer, esophageal cancer, and cancers of the small intestine. Potentially, intake of blueberries may lower the risks of these types of cancers.

"IF YOU KEEP GOOD FOOD IN YOUR FRIDGE, YOU WILL EAT GOOD FOOD"

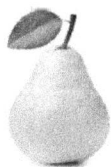

PEARS

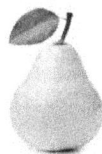

NUTRITION FACTS

VITAMINS – Vitamin C (4.3mg),
Thiamin (0.012mg), Riboflavin (0.026mg),
Niacin (0.161mg), Vitamin B6 (0.029mg),
Folate (7µg), Vitamin A (1µg),
Vitamin E (0.12mg) and Vitamin K (4.4µg)

MINERALS – Calcium (9mg),
Iron (0.18mg), Magnesium (7mg),
Phosphorus (12mg), Potassium (116mg),
Sodium (1mg) and Zinc (0.1mg).

[USDA national nutrient database, 2015]

Nutrient	Value per 100g
Energy	57kcal
Protein	0.36g
Fat	0.14g
Carbohydrate	15.23g
Fibre	3.1g
Sugar	9.75g

HEALTH BENEFITS

☆ **Healthier digestive tract and prevents constipation**

☆ **Reduces pressure and inflammation in the colon**

☆ **Helps lower blood pressure and cholesterol**

☆ **Lower risk of developing diabetes and keeps blood sugar stable**

☆ **Antioxidant benefits**

☆ **Anti-inflammatory benefits**

The phytonutrients found in pears provide us with antioxidants as well as anti-inflammatory benefits. As a result, the consumption of pears has now been associated with decreased risk of several common chronic diseases that begin with chronic inflammation and excessive oxidative stress.

The good source of fibre content in pears help protect us from development of type 2 diabetes as well heart disease. This is due to the helpful combination of both soluble and insoluble fibre in this fruit. In addition to their fibre content, however, pears have other ways of helping to protect us against these diseases.

Intake of pears can also reduce the risk of various types of cancers. The fibre content from pear can bind together not only with bile acids as a whole, but also with a special group of bile acids called secondary bile acids. Excessive amounts of secondary bile acids in the intestine can increase our risk of colorectal cancer (as well as other intestinal problems). By binding together with secondary bile acids, pear fibres can help decrease their concentration in the intestine and lower our risk of cancer development. This also the case with stomach cancer. Here the key focus has not been on pear fibre, however, but on pear phytonutrients, especially cinnamic acids (including coumaric acid, ferulic acid, and 5-caffeoylquinic acid).

Consumption of pears can also reduce the risk of a third type of cancer known as esophageal cancer (specifically, esophageal squamous cell carcinoma, or ESCC).

Increased fibre content has also been shown to lower blood pressure and cholesterol levels. It prevents constipation and promotes regularity for a healthy digestive tract.

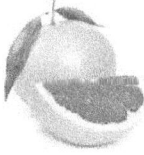

GRAPEFRUIT

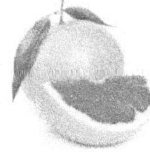

NUTRITION FACTS

VITAMINS – Vitamin C (34.4mg),
Thiamin (0.036mg), Riboflavin (0.02mg),
Niacin (0.25mg), Vitamin B6 (0.042mg),
Folate (10µg), Vitamin A (46µg) and
Vitamin E (0.13mg)

MINERALS – Calcium (12mg),
Iron (0.09mg), Magnesium (8mg),
Phosphorus (8mg), Potassium (139mg) and
Zinc (0.07mg).

[USDA national nutrient database, 2015]

Nutrient	Value per 100g
Energy	32kcal
Protein	0.63g
Fat	0.1g
Carbohydrate	8.08g
Fibre	1.1g
Sugar	6.98g

HEALTH BENEFITS

☆ **Helps prevent strokes**

☆ **Reduces blood pressure**

☆ **Cardiovascular benefits**

☆ **Anti-cancer**

☆ **Prevents constipation and promote regularity for a healthy digestive tract**

☆ **Great snack to have on hand to prevent dehydration**

☆ **Helps fight skin damage**

☆ **Anti-asthma**

Increased consumption of grapefruit has been shown to decrease the risk of obesity, diabetes, heart disease and overall mortality while promoting a healthy complexion, increased energy, and overall lower weight.

According to the American Heart Association, ischemic stroke risk in women could be lowered by eating higher amounts of citrus fruits like oranges and grapefruit.

The powerful nutrient combination of fibre, potassium, lycopene, vitamin C and choline in grapefruit all help to maintain a healthy heart. Increasing potassium intake is also important for lowering blood pressure because of its powerful vasodilation effects.

Reduced risk of stroke, protection against loss of muscle mass, preservation of bone mineral density and reduction in the formation of kidney stones are all associated with the high content of potassium present in grapefruits.

With grapefruit's excellent source of the strong antioxidant vitamin C as well as other antioxidants, it can help combat the formation of free radicals known to cause cancer. The intake of lycopene has been linked with a decreased risk of prostate cancer and beta-carotene have been shown in particular to lower the risk of esophageal cancer.

Due to the water and fibre content found in grapefruit, constipation can be prevented and regularity for a healthy digestive tract can be promoted.

As one of the most hydrating fruits in the world made up of 91% water (just below watermelon) and full of important electrolytes, grapefruit is a great snack to have on hand to prevent dehydration.

When grapefruit is eaten in its natural form (in fresh produce as opposed to supplement form) or applied topically, the antioxidant vitamin C present, can help to fight skin damage caused by the sun and pollution, reduce wrinkles and improve overall skin texture. Vitamin C plays a vital role in the formation of collagen, the main support system of skin and can lower the risk of developing asthma. Hydration and vitamin A are also crucial for healthy looking skin, both of which grapefruits can provide.

However, consuming grapefruit in large amounts should be avoided as it may put us at higher risk of melanoma, the deadliest form of skin cancer.

"YOUR GOOD HEALTH IS YOUR GREATEST WEALTH"

KIWIFRUIT

NUTRITION FACTS

VITAMINS – Vitamin C (92.7mg), Thiamin (0.027mg), Riboflavin (0.025mg), Niacin (0.341mg), Vitamin B6 (0.063mg), Folate (25µg), Vitamin A (4µg), Vitamin E (1.46mg) and Vitamin K (40.3µg)

MINERALS – Calcium (34mg), Iron (0.31mg), Magnesium (17mg), Phosphorus (34mg), Potassium (312mg), Sodium (3mg) and Zinc (0.14mg).

[USDA national nutrient database, 2015]

Nutrient	Value per 100g
Energy	61kcal
Protein	1.14g
Fat	0.52g
Carbohydrate	14.66g
Fibre	3g
Sugar	8.99g

HEALTH BENEFITS

☆ **Cardiovascular benefits**

☆ **Better sleep**

☆ **Anti-aging**

☆ **Anti-asthma**

☆ **Prevents constipation**

☆ **Antioxidant benefits**

☆ **Helps lower blood pressure and cholesterol**

Kiwifruit can offer a great deal more than an exotic tropical flair in your fruit salad. The phytonutrient present in kiwifruit has been found to protect DNA in the nucleus of human cells from oxygen-related damage.

Kiwifruit is an excellent source of vitamin C. This nutrient is the primary water-soluble antioxidant in the body, neutralizing free radicals that can cause damage to cells and lead to problems such as inflammation and cancer. In fact, adequate intake of vitamin C has been shown to be helpful in reducing the severity of conditions like osteoarthritis, rheumatoid arthritis, and asthma, and for preventing conditions such as colon cancer, atherosclerosis, and diabetic heart disease. And since vitamin C is necessary for the healthy function of the immune system, it may be useful for preventing recurrent ear infections in people who suffer from them. Eating fruits rich in vitamin C such as kiwifruit may confer a significant protective effect against respiratory symptoms associated with asthma such as wheezing.

The increased fibre content found in kiwifruit has also been shown to be useful for a number of conditions such as reducing high cholesterol levels, which may reduce the risk of heart disease and heart attack. Fibre is also good for binding and removing toxins from the colon, which is helpful for preventing colon cancer. In addition, fibre-rich foods, like kiwifruit, are good for keeping the blood sugar levels of diabetic patients under control.

Enjoying just a couple of kiwifruit each day may significantly lower your risk for blood clots and reduce the amount of fats (triglycerides) in your blood, therefore helping to protect cardiovascular health.

Unlike aspirin, which also helps to reduce blood clotting but has side effects such as inflammation and bleeding in the intestinal tract, the effects of regular kiwi consumption are all beneficial. Kiwifruit is an excellent source of vitamin C, and polyphenols, and a good source of potassium, all of which may function individually or in concert to protect the blood vessels and heart.

The high potassium content in kiwifruit can help undo the effects of sodium in the body. It is possible that a low potassium intake is just as big of a risk factor in developing high blood pressure as a high sodium intake.

Collagen which supports the skin is reliant on vitamin C as an essential nutrient that works in our bodies as an antioxidant to help prevent damage caused by the sun, pollution and smoke, smooth wrinkles and improve overall skin texture. Thus kiwifruit being very beneficial to a healthier looking complexion.

According to a study on the effects of kiwifruit consumption on sleep quality in adults with sleep problems, it was found that kiwi consumption may improve sleep onset, duration and efficiency in adults with self-reported sleep disturbances.

Several studies have shown that kiwifruit may have a mild laxative effect and could be used as a dietary supplement especially for elderly individuals experiencing constipation. Regular consumption of kiwifruit was shown to promote bulkier, softer and more frequent stool production.

"EAT GOOD, FEEL GOOD, LOOK GOOD"

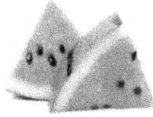

WATERMELON

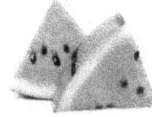

NUTRITION FACTS

VITAMINS – Vitamin C (8.1mg), Thiamin (0.033mg), Riboflavin (0.021mg), Niacin (0.178mg), Vitamin B6 (0.045mg), Folate (3µg), Vitamin A (28µg), Vitamin E (0.05mg) and Vitamin K (0.1µg)

MINERALS – Calcium (7mg), Iron (0.24mg), Magnesium (10mg), Phosphorus (11mg), Potassium (112mg), Sodium (1mg) and Zinc (0.1mg).

[USDA national nutrient database, 2015]

Nutrient	Value per 100g
Energy	30kcal
Protein	0.61g
Fat	0.15g
Carbohydrate	7.55g
Fibre	0.4g
Sugar	6.2g

HEALTH BENEFITS

☆ **Anti-asthma**

☆ **Anti-aging**

☆ **Lowers blood pressure**

☆ **Anti-cancer**

☆ **Helps with muscle soreness**

☆ **Anti-inflammation**

☆ **Helps with constipation and regulates normal digestion**

☆ **Keeps you hydrated**

The high nutrient of vitamin C in watermelons help prevent developing asthma.

Studies have shown that watermelon extract supplementation reduced ankle blood pressure, brachial blood pressure and carotid wave reflection in obese middle-aged adults with pre-hypertension or stage 1 hypertension and that watermelon extract improved arterial function.

The excellent source of vitamin C has also shown to help combat the formation of free radicals known to cause cancer.

Lycopene intake, also found in watermelon have shown to help protect against heart diseases and has been linked with a decreased risk of prostate cancer prevention.

Due to the water and fibre content in watermelons, it has shown to help prevent constipation and promote regularity for a healthy digestive tract.

As watermelons are made up of 92% water and full of important electrolytes, it is a great snack to have on hand during the hot summer months to prevent dehydration of the body.

Another versatile nutrient found in watermelons is choline that aids our bodies in sleep, muscle movement, learning and memory. Choline also helps to maintain the structure of cellular membranes, aids in the transmission of nerve impulses, assists in the absorption of fat and reduces chronic inflammation.

Muscle soreness has been shown to be improved by intake of watermelon and watermelon juice thus improves recovery time following exercise in athletes.

Watermelon is also fantastic for your skin because it contains vitamin A, a nutrient required for sebum production which also keeps hair moisturized. Vitamin A is generally required for the growth of all bodily tissues. Watermelon also contributes to overall hydration, which is vital for having healthy looking skin and hair.

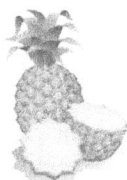

PINEAPPLE

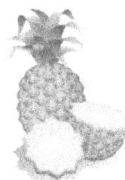

NUTRITION FACTS

VITAMINS – Vitamin C (47.8mg), Thiamin (0.079mg), Riboflavin (0.032mg), Niacin (0.5mg), Vitamin B6 (0.112mg), Folate (18µg), Vitamin A (3µg), Vitamin E (0.02mg) and Vitamin K (0.7µg)

MINERALS – Calcium (13mg), Iron (0.29mg), Magnesium (12mg), Phosphorus (8mg), Potassium (109mg), Sodium (1mg) and Zinc (0.12mg).

[USDA national nutrient database, 2015]

Nutrient	Value per 100g
Energy	50kcal
Protein	0.54g
Fat	0.12g
Carbohydrate	13.12g
Fibre	1.4g
Sugar	9.85g

HEALTH BENEFITS

☆ **Anti-asthma**

☆ **Anti-cancer**

☆ **Lowers blood pressure**

☆ **Improves fertility**

☆ **Prevents diabetes**

☆ **Antioxidant benefits**

☆ **Fights skin damage**

☆ **Cardiovascular benefits**

☆ **Healing and inflammation benefits**

Beta-carotene, found in pineapple help lower the risks for developing asthma as well as playing a role in protecting against prostate cancer.

Increased potassium content helps with lowering blood pressure. And in general associated with decreased risk of dying from all causes.

The increased amounts of vitamin C found in pineapples can help combat the formation of free radicals known to cause cancer.

High fibre intakes from all fruits and vegetables are associated with a lowered risk of colorectal cancer.

Studies have shown that type 1 diabetics who consume high-fibre diets have lower blood glucose levels and type 2 diabetics may have improved blood sugar, lipids and insulin levels. One medium pineapple provides about 13 grams of fibre.

Pineapples, because of their high levels of fibre and water content, help to prevent constipation and promote regularity and a healthy digestive tract.

Fertility has also been shown to be improved by consumption of pineapples. Because free radicals also can damage the reproductive system, foods with high antioxidant activity like pineapples that battle free radicals are recommended for those trying to conceive. The antioxidants in pineapple such as vitamins C, beta-carotene and the vitamins and minerals and copper, zinc and folate have properties that affect both male and female fertility.

The enzyme bromelain, found in pineapples, can reduce swelling, bruising, healing time, and pain associated with injury and surgical intervention.

The combination of fibre, potassium and vitamin C content in pineapple all help prevent cardiovascular diseases.

High potassium intakes are also associated with a reduced risk of stroke, protection against loss of muscle mass, preservation of bone mineral density and reduction in the formation of kidney stones.

The antioxidant vitamin C, when eaten in its natural form (as in a pineapple) or applied topically, can help to fight skin damage caused by the sun and pollution, reduce wrinkles and improve overall skin texture giving a more healthier complexion.

"THINK OF WHAT YOU PUT IN YOUR MOUTH, THAT'S WHAT HEALTHY EATING IS ALL ABOUT"

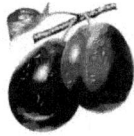

PLUM

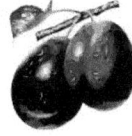

NUTRITION FACTS

VITAMINS – Vitamin C (9.5mg), Thiamin (0.028mg), Riboflavin (0.026mg), Niacin (0.417mg), Vitamin B6 (0.029mg), Folate (5µg), Vitamin A (17µg), Vitamin E (0.26mg) and Vitamin K (6.4µg)

MINERALS – Calcium (6mg), Iron (0.17mg), Magnesium (7mg), Phosphorus (16mg), Potassium (157mg)and Zinc (0.1mg).

[USDA national nutrient database, 2015]

Nutrient	Value per 100g
Energy	46kcal
Protein	0.7g
Fat	0.28g
Carbohydrate	11.42g
Fibre	1.4g
Sugar	9.92g

HEALTH BENEFITS

☆ **Antioxidant benefits**

☆ **Anti-cancer**

☆ **Anti-aging**

☆ **Prevents constipation and regulates a healthier digestive tract**

☆ **Beneficial in pregnancy**

☆ **Cardiovascular benefits**

Plums are packed with an immense range of phenols and flavonoids, which provide us with several health benefits.

Plums contain vitamin C and phytonutrients such as lutein, cryptoxanthin, zeaxanthin, neochlorogenic and chlorogenic acid. These components possess effective antioxidant qualities which help in preventing the damage caused by oxygen radicals called superoxide anion radicals. The phenols present in plums also extend their protective effect on the essential fats in the neurons and cell membranes against any injuries caused by oxidative stress.

The flavonoids and phenolic components present in plums exert anti-obesity and anti-inflammatory effects on the different bodily cells, including the fat cells, and they also help in preventing obesity-related problems such as cholesterol disorders, diabetes and cardiovascular diseases.

Flavonoids such as caffeic acid and rutin that are both present in plums help in inhibiting the deterioration of bone tissues and prevent diseases such as osteoporosis in postmenopausal women. Consumption of dried plums exerts anabolic and anti-resorptive actions, which aid in maintaining healthy bones. Polyphenols, along with the potassium content present in dried plums, encourage the formation of bones, enhances bone density and prevents bone loss caused by ovarian hormone deficiency.

Plums exert anti-hyperglycemic effects and help in combating diabetes. Studies have shown that the consumption of plum extracts aids in the reduction of blood glucose and levels of triglyceride in the body. The flavonoids present in plums exert protective effects against insulin resistance and help to enhance insulin sensitivity in the body.

The high content in fibre along with the components sorbitol and isatin, which help in regulating the digestive system. According to research studies, dried plums or prunes are more effective in treating digestive disorders such as constipation. Sorbitol and isatin have a laxative effect and encourage the secretion of fluids in the bowels and promote the efficient flushing of waste through the colon.

Flavonoids present in plum juice have shown to be effective in providing protection against age-related cognitive impairment. The beneficial phytonutrients present in plums help in reducing the inflammation in the neurological areas to improve learning and memory functions. Regular consumption of plums also helps in preventing age-related neurodegenerative disorders such as Alzheimer's and Parkinson's diseases.

The intake of plums helps prevent cardiovascular diseases. Regular intake of dried plums helps in promoting fluidity of blood in the arteries. This protective effect aids in the prevention of various cardiac disorders, including the development of atherosclerosis and the reduction in chances for heart attacks and strokes.

The immune system is strengthened by the consumption of plums and by the presence of high vitamin C content. It promotes the body's resistance against various infections and inflammation.

Vitamin B6, found in plums, helps in the transmission of nerve signals and aids in the smooth functioning of the nervous system. Plums also help in the normal growth of the brain and assist in the formation of mood influencing hormones. Tryptophan, an amino acid present in plums, helps in the production of the neurotransmitter serotonin, which plays an important role in the sleep, appetite and concentration.

Dried plums or prunes help in preventing hypercholesterolemia and hyperlipidemia. The fibre content present in plums also adds to the protective effect of the heart by reducing LDL cholesterol and helping to elevate the levels of HDL cholesterol (good cholesterol).

Plums contains essential iron and copper which assists in the formation of red blood cells and facilitates blood purification and healthy circulation. The copper in plums acts as an antioxidant and is essential for nerve health and aids in the formation of collagen. Consumption of copper-rich plums also helps in the absorption of iron and prevents various diseases such as anaemia and osteoarthritis.

Plums are beneficial during pregnancy, due to the abundance of numerous vitamins and minerals. These beneficial components are vital for eye-sight, development of bones and tissues, and cellular health for the mother and the growing baby. The fibre content aids in preventing constipation and improves digestion. The inclusion of plums as a part of balanced diet helps in fighting various infections and maintains overall health. However, one should be careful regarding the choice of commercially available plum juices as they might contain high amounts of sugar.

Plum extracts have been proven beneficial in the treatment of cancer. Plums are rich in antioxidants and phytonutrients, including chlorogenic acid and neo-chlorogenic acid which have a curative effect against breast cancer cells, without harming the normal healthy cells of the body.

The rich source of vitamin C in plums, along with other antioxidants, help to maintain healthy and radiant skin complexion. The consumption of plums helps in reducing dark spots and wrinkles due to the presence of anti-aging nutrients.

Plums contains vitamin A and beta-carotene, which are beneficial in maintaining healthy eye sight and preventing age-related macular degeneration. The carotenoids, lutein and zeaxanthin present in plums reside in the macular tissues of the retina and provide protection against the damage caused by ultraviolet (UV) radiation.

Plums contain vitamin K, which helps in normal clotting of the blood and promotes bone health. Deficiency of vitamin K in the body can result in excessive blood loss and other health concerns such as weak bones.

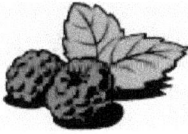

RASPBERRIES

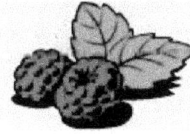

NUTRITION FACTS

VITAMINS – Vitamin C (26.2mg),
Thiamin (0.032mg), Riboflavin (0.038mg),
Niacin (0.598mg), Vitamin B6 (0.055mg),
Folate (21µg), Vitamin A (2µg),
Vitamin E (0.87mg) and Vitamin K (7.8µg)

MINERALS – Calcium (25mg),
Iron (0.69mg), Magnesium (22mg),
Phosphorus (29mg), Potassium (151mg),
Sodium (1mg) and Zinc (0.42mg).

[USDA national nutrient database, 2015]

Nutrient	Value per 100g
Energy	52kcal
Protein	1.2g
Fat	0.65g
Carbohydrate	11.94g
Fibre	6.5g
Sugar	4.42g

HEALTH BENEFITS

☆ **Anti-inflammatory benefits**

☆ **Cardiovascular benefits**

☆ **Anti-cancer**

☆ **Diabetic prevention**

☆ **Improves digestive system**

☆ **Eye health benefits**

Flavonoid-rich foods like raspberries result in a lower risk of cardiovascular diseases.

One flavonoid in particular, anthocyanins, have been shown to suppress inflammation that may lead to cardiovascular disease. The high polyphenol content in raspberries may also reduce the risk of cardiovascular disease by preventing platelet build up and reducing blood pressure via anti-inflammatory mechanisms.

The potassium in raspberries help prevent ischemic heart disease.

Raspberries contain powerful antioxidants that work against free radicals, inhibiting tumour growth and decreasing inflammation in the body. Those same potent polyphenols that protect against heart disease also help prevent cancer, including esophageal, lung, mouth, pharynx, endometrial, pancreatic, prostate and colon cancer.

The high fibre content in raspberries help manage diabetes in diabetic individuals.

The combination of both fibre and water content in raspberries help to prevent constipation and maintain a healthy digestive tract.

Raspberries are also high in vitamin C which have shown to help keep eyes healthy by providing protection against UV light damage.

Raspberries also contain the antioxidant zeaxanthin, which filters out harmful blue light rays and is thought to play a protective role in eye health and possibly prevent damage from macular degeneration.

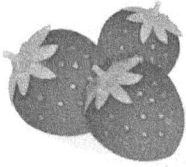

STRAWBERRIES

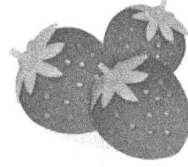

NUTRITION FACTS

VITAMINS – Vitamin C (58.8mg), Thiamin (0.024mg), Riboflavin (0.022mg), Niacin (0.386mg), Vitamin B6 (0.047mg), Folate (24µg), Vitamin A (1µg), Vitamin E (0.29mg) and Vitamin K (2.2µg)

MINERALS – Calcium (16mg), Iron (0.41mg), Magnesium (13mg), Phosphorus (24mg), Potassium (153mg), Sodium (1mg) and Zinc (0.14mg).

[USDA national nutrient database, 2015]

Nutrient	Value per 100g
Energy	32kcal
Protein	0.67g
Fat	0.3g
Carbohydrate	7.68g
Fibre	2g
Sugar	4.89g

HEALTH BENEFITS

☆ **Cardiovascular benefits**

☆ **Prevents strokes**

☆ **Anti-cancer**

☆ **Anti-asthma**

☆ **Prevents constipation and helps regularity of digestive tract**

☆ **Beneficial in pregnancy**

☆ **Lowers blood pressure**

☆ **Prevents depression**

Regular consumption of anthocyanins, a class of flavonoids found in strawberries, can reduce the risk of a heart attacks.

The flavonoid quercetin, contained in strawberries, is a natural anti-inflammatory that appears to reduce the risk of atherosclerosis.

The high polyphenol content in strawberries may also reduce the risk of cardiovascular disease by preventing platelet build-up and reducing blood pressure via anti-inflammatory mechanisms.

The fibre and potassium in strawberries also support heart health.

The antioxidants quercetin, kaempferol, and anthocyanins have all been shown to reduce the formation of harmful blood clots associated with strokes. High potassium intakes have also been linked with a reduced risk of stroke.

Strawberries contain powerful antioxidants that work against free radicals, inhibiting tumour growth and decreasing inflammation in the body.

Due to their high potassium content, strawberries are recommended to those with high blood pressure to help undo the effects of sodium in the body. A low potassium intake is just as big of a risk factor in developing high blood pressure as a high sodium intake.

The high levels of fibre content in strawberries is essential for minimizing constipation.

Because of the anti-inflammatory effects of quercetin, consuming strawberries may help to alleviate symptoms of allergies including runny nose, watery eyes and hives. Prevention of asthma is lower with a high intake of certain nutrients such as vitamin C present in strawberries.

Strawberries are a low glycemic index food and high in fibre, which helps to regulate blood sugar and keep it stable by avoiding extreme highs and lows.

Adequate folic acid intake present in strawberries is essential for pregnant women to protect against neural tube defects in infants.

Folate may also help with depression by preventing an excess of homocysteine from forming in the body, which can prevent blood and other nutrients from reaching the brain. Excess homocysteine interferes with the production of the feel-good hormones serotonin, dopamine, and norepinephrine, which regulate not only mood, but sleep and appetite as well.

"WATCH WHAT YOU EAT TODAY, SO TOMORROW YOU CAN KEEP DISEASES AWAY"

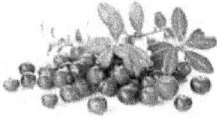

CRANBERRIES

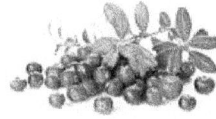

NUTRITION FACTS

VITAMINS – Vitamin C (14mg), Thiamin (0.012mg), Riboflavin (0.02mg), Niacin (0.101mg), Vitamin B6 (0.057mg), Folate (1μg), Vitamin A (3μg), Vitamin E (1.32mg) and Vitamin K (5μg)

MINERALS – Calcium (8mg), Iron (0.23mg), Magnesium (6mg), Phosphorus (11mg), Potassium (80mg), Sodium (2mg) and Zinc (0.09mg).

[USDA national nutrient database, 2015]

Nutrient	Value per 100g
Energy	46kcal
Protein	0.46g
Fat	0.13g
Carbohydrate	11.97g
Fibre	3.6g
Sugar	4.27g

HEALTH BENEFITS

☆ **Prevents urinary tract infection**

☆ **Cardiovascular benefits**

☆ **Anti-cancer**

☆ **Oral health benefits**

The high level of proanthocyanidins (PACs) in cranberries helps reduce the adhesion of certain bacteria to the urinary tract walls, in turn fighting off infections.

Polyphenols in cranberries may reduce the risk of cardiovascular disease by preventing platelet build-up and reducing blood pressure via anti-inflammatory mechanisms.

Studies have shown that cranberries are beneficial in slowing tumor progression and have shown positive effects against prostate, liver, ovarian, breast and colon cancers.

The same proanthocyanidins in cranberries that help prevent urinal tract infections may also benefit oral health by preventing bacteria from binding to teeth. Cranberries may also be beneficial in preventing gum disease.

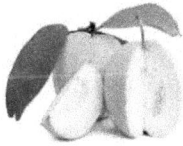

GUAVA

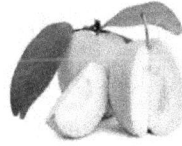

NUTRITION FACTS

VITAMINS – Vitamin C (228.3mg),
Thiamin (0.067mg), Riboflavin (0.04mg),
Niacin (1.084mg), Vitamin B6 (0.11mg),
Folate (49µg), Vitamin A (31µg),
Vitamin E (0.73mg) and Vitamin K (2.6µg)

MINERALS – Calcium (18mg),
Iron (0.26mg), Magnesium (22mg),
Phosphorus (40mg), Potassium (417mg),
Sodium (2mg) and Zinc (0.23mg).

[USDA national nutrient database, 2015]

Nutrient	Value per 100g
Energy	68kcal
Protein	2.55g
Fat	0.95g
Carbohydrate	14.32g
Fibre	5.4g
Sugar	8.92g

HEALTH BENEFITS

☆ **May help to prevent diabetes**

☆ **Anti-cancer**

☆ **Healthy vision**

☆ **Reduces symptoms of diarrhea & dysentery**

☆ **Prevents constipation**

☆ **Helps regulate thyroid metabolism**

☆ **Cognitive benefits**

☆ **Relieves coughs and colds**

☆ **Anti-aging**

☆ **Reduces cholesterol and high blood pressure**

Guava is and rich in vitamins, proteins and minerals, but it has no cholesterol and a low number of digestible carbohydrates. It is a is very filling snack and satisfies the appetite very easily.

Consumption of guava can help patients who suffer from diabetes. The high level of dietary fibre in guava helps to regulate the absorption of sugar by the body, which decreases the chances of major spikes and drops in insulin and glucose in the body. Various research studies have shown that the intake of guava in our diets can help prevent the appearance of type-2 diabetes.

Guavas are an extremely good source of vitamin A, which is well known as for benefits in vision Therefore consumption can help slow down the appearance of cataracts, macular degeneration, and general health of the eyes. It can not only prevent degradation of eyesight, but even an improvement in eyesight once it has begun to degrade.

Intake of guavas play an important role in regulating thyroid metabolism, due to its good source of copper, by helping to control hormone production and absorption. The thyroid gland is one of the most important glands in the body for regulating hormones and organ system function, so guava can help balance your health in many ways.

The most important benefits of guavas is its ability to inhibit the growth and metastasis of cancerous cells, especially prostate cancer, breast cancer, and oral cancers.

Finally, the naturally high levels of vitamin C in guavas, which are four times higher than the levels found in oranges provides the immune system a huge boost in antioxidants. Antioxidants are the major lines of defence against the proliferation of free radicals in the body, which are one of the main causes of serious conditions like cancer and heart disease. Therefore, adding guava to your diet has numerous ways in which it helps you stay healthy and cancer free.

The very high content of fibre in guavas help the formation of healthy bowel movements, and aid the body in retaining water and thoroughly cleaning your intestines and excretory system. Thus it is a great fruit for preventing constipation.

Eating raw guava helps your mouth feel refreshed as well as helping to loosen your bowels and reduce symptoms of diarrhoea. Guavas are alkaline in nature and have disinfectant and anti-bacterial properties, thus helping to cure dysentery by inhibiting microbial growth and removing extra mucus from the intestines. Also other nutrients in guava such as vitamin C, potassium and carotenoids, strengthen and tone the digestive system as well as disinfecting it. Guava is also beneficial in treating

The presence of niacin and B6 vitamins in guavas is also very beneficial. Niacin can increase blood flow and stimulate cognitive function. Vitamin B6 is a great nutrient for brain and nerve function. Therefore, eating guava can help you increase brain function and sharpen your focus.

Guava juice a decoction of guava-leaves is very helpful in relieving coughs and colds by reducing mucus, disinfecting the respiratory tract, throat and lungs, and inhibiting microbial activity with its astringent properties. Guava has one of the highest quantities of vitamin C and iron among fruits, and both are proven to be preventive against colds and viral infections. However ripe guava should be avoided by people who are suffering from cough and cold, as it can exacerbate the problem, and one should also avoid drinking water immediately after eating guava as it can lead to a sore throat.

Guava is also known to improve skin conditions as it is rich in vitamin A, B, C and potassium which are good antioxidants and detoxifiers, which keep your skin glowing and free from signs of premature aging, wrinkles and other dermal disorders.

Guava has known to reduce cholesterol in the blood and prevents it from thickening, thereby maintaining the fluidity of blood and reducing blood pressure due to its very rich fibre and hypoglycemic nature.

VEGETABLES

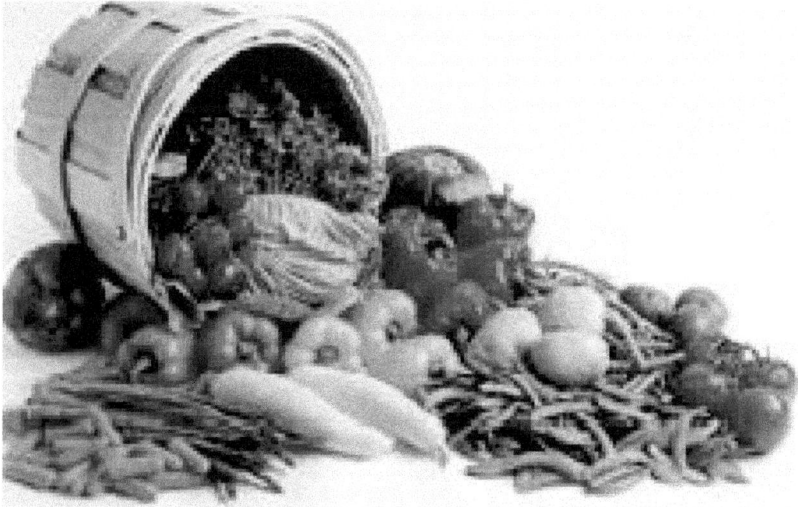

HEALTH BENEFITS OF VEGETABLES

Vegetables have a lot of vitamins, minerals, fibre, and phytochemicals. They are low in calories, fat and sugar. The differently coloured vegetables, green, orange, red and yellow, have different phytochemicals which act as antioxidants that help to eliminate free radicals from the body. These free radicals are the main causative molecules for inducing diseases like cancer, high blood pressure, diabetes, eye disease like cataract, and age related macular degeneration. Also phytochemicals delay aging and wrinkling of the skin. Micro elements in vegetables are needed to build new tissues, bones, muscles, blood cells, enzymes, hormones, and DNA. These elements are needed for all metabolic activities like nerve function, respiration, muscle contraction, enzyme activity and blood clotting.

Vegetables have a lot of soluble and insoluble fibre such as cellulose, mucilage, and pectin. These absorb excess water in the colon and retain moisture in the faecal matter, help in easy digestion, the easy movement of digested food, and help to reduce constipation, thus protecting the mucous membrane of the colon by decreasing the exposure time to toxic substances. Sufficient fibre in food gives protection from colon cancer and constipation. High fibre in foods helps to control diabetes, obesity and cholesterol levels of blood by decreasing its absorption in the colon. Recent scientific studies have shown that low calorie, nutrient rich foods help the human body to develop immunity and strength to fight against disease.

Most of the antioxidants in vegetables help to reduce cancer in the colon, lungs, breast, prostate and pancreas.

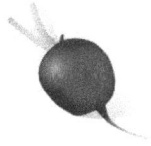

BEETROOT

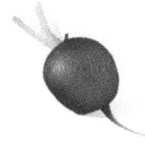

NUTRITION FACTS

VITAMINS – Vitamin C (4.9mg), Thiamin (0.031mg), Riboflavin (0.04mg), Niacin (0.334mg), Vitamin B6 (0.067mg), Folate (109μg), Vitamin A (2μg), Vitamin E (0.04mg) and Vitamin K (0.2μg)

MINERALS – Calcium (16mg), Iron (0.8mg), Magnesium (23mg), Phosphorus (40mg), Potassium (325mg), Sodium (78mg) and Zinc (0.35mg).

[USDA national nutrient database, 2015]

Nutrient	Value per 100g
Energy	43kcal
Protein	1.61g
Fat	0.17g
Carbohydrate	9.56g
Fibre	2.8g
Sugar	6.76g

HEALTH BENEFITS

☆ **Cardiovascular benefits**

☆ **Anti-inflammatory**

☆ **Slows down the progression of dementia in older adults**

☆ **Antioxidant benefits**

☆ **Prevents constipation and promotes regularity for a healthy digestive tract**

☆ **Beneficial for diabetics as it lowers glucose levels**

☆ **Essential nutrients during pregnancy**

Recent research has shown that the high nitrate content in beetroot is absorbed by the intestine and is converted to nitric oxide in the body. This nitric oxide dilates blood vessels and reduces blood pressure. Nitric oxide helps in increasing blood supply to the brain and improves brain function. Research has shown that drinking juice from beetroot can improve oxygenation to the brain, slowing the progression of dementia in older adults. Blood flow to certain areas of the brain decrease with age and leads to a decline in cognition and possible dementia. Consuming beetroot juice as part of a high nitrate diet can improve the blood flow and oxygenation to these areas that are lacking.

Betanine in beetroot enhances the production of serotonin, a natural mood lifter in the body; beetroot can make you happy.

Iron and folate are essential for the formation of red blood cells and haemoglobin. This helps to reduce the anaemic condition of the body. Young beetroot leaves are a better source of iron. Recent discoveries found that folate is essential for pregnant mothers; folate is involved in the development of the spinal cord during first three months of pregnancy.

Vitamins and minerals in beetroot help in the production of new body cells and boosting the immune system.

Betacyanine in beetroot is an antioxidant which helps detox the liver, eliminates toxins and protects liver cells' DNA. Antioxidants help to remove free radicals and protect the cells from the risk of non-communicable diseases.

Calcium is important for muscular and skeletal health.

Research has shown that drinking beetroot juice in the morning helps to reduce high blood pressure.

Lutein helps the health of the retina of eye, and reduces age related eye defects.

Beetroot has been shown to be beneficial in diabetic patients as it contains an antioxidant known as alpha-lipoic acid, which has been shown to lower glucose levels, increase insulin sensitivity and prevent oxidative stress-induced changes.

Due to the high fibre content, beetroot helps to prevent constipation and promote regularity for a healthy digestive tract.

Choline is a very important and versatile nutrient in beetroot that helps with sleep, muscle movement, learning and memory. The structure of the cellular membrane is also maintained by the help of choline. Choline, aids in the transmission of nerve impulses, assists in the absorption of fat and reduces chronic inflammation.

"WANT TO LOOK GOOD AND FEEL GREAT? HAVE GRAINS AND VEGGIES ON YOUR PLATE"

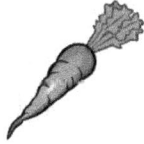

CARROT

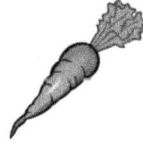

NUTRITION FACTS

VITAMINS – Vitamin C (5.9mg), Thiamin (0.066mg), Riboflavin (0.058mg), Niacin (0.983mg), Vitamin B6 (0.138mg), Folate (19µg), Vitamin A (835µg), Vitamin E (0.66mg) and Vitamin K (13.2µg)

MINERALS – Calcium (33mg), Iron (0.3mg), Magnesium (12mg), Phosphorus (35mg), Potassium (320mg), Sodium (69mg) and Zinc (0.24mg).

[USDA national nutrient database, 2015]

Nutrient	Value per 100g
Energy	41kcal
Protein	0.93g
Fat	0.24g
Carbohydrate	9.58g
Fibre	2.8g
Sugar	4.74g

HEALTH BENEFITS

☆ **Anti-cancer**

☆ **Good vision**

☆ **Antioxidants benefits**

☆ **Regulate blood sugar**

☆ **Delay the effects of aging**

☆ **Improve immune function**

☆ **Prevents constipation and facilitates easy bowl movements**

Carrots are rich in beta carotene, which is converted to vitamin A in the body. This vitamin A is necessary for good vision, reproduction, and the maintenance of epithelial integrity, growth and development. Vitamin A prevents cataracts and is good for skin disorders. Vitamin A and the antioxidants in carrots protect the skin from sun damage

Vitamin A prevents premature wrinkling, as well as dry uneven skin tone. It also flushes out the toxins from the body and reduces bile and fat in the liver.

Vitamin C helps the body to maintain healthy connective tissue, teeth and gums. It reduces the harmful effects of free radicals on the cells.

The high level of fibre in carrots helps in lowering blood sugar and cholesterol levels because the soluble fibres in carrots bind with bile acids and LDL. Fibre reduces constipation and facilitates easy bowl movements, which prevents cancer risk in the intestine.

High levels of beta carotene act as a powerful antioxidant that helps in protecting the body from free radical damage. Lutein helps in protecting the eyes from age related eye defects in elderly people. The antioxidants in carrots fight against cancer by destroying cancerous cells in tumours.

There are high levels of minerals in carrots. Potassium is an important component of body fluids that helps maintain the heart rate and blood pressure by countering the effects of sodium.

Recent research has found that falcarinol in carrots acts as an antioxidant that reduces the risk of lung cancer, colon cancer, and breast cancer.

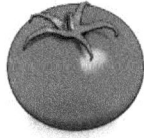

TOMATO

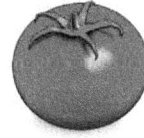

NUTRITION FACTS

VITAMINS – Vitamin C (13.7mg),
Thiamin (0.037mg), Riboflavin (0.019mg),
Niacin (0.594mg), Vitamin B6 (0.08mg),
Folate (15µg), Vitamin A (42µg),
Vitamin E (0.54mg) and Vitamin K (7.9µg)

MINERALS – Calcium (10mg),
Iron (0.27mg), Magnesium (11mg),
Phosphorus (24mg), Potassium (237mg),
Sodium (5mg) and Zinc (0.17mg).

[USDA national nutrient database, 2015]

Nutrient	Value per 100g
Energy	18kcal
Protein	0.88g
Fat	0.2g
Carbohydrate	3.89g
Fibre	1.2g
Sugar	2.63g

HEALTH BENEFITS

☆ **Antioxidant benefits**

☆ **Anti-cancer**

☆ **Cardiovascular benefits**

☆ **Beneficial in pregnancy**

☆ **Helps prevent depression**

☆ **Prevents constipation and facilitates easy bowl movements**

☆ **Regulates blood sugar and glucose levels**

☆ **Anti-aging**

Tomato is a lycopene rich fruit. It has been found that lycopene reduces the risk of stomach, mouth, pharynx, colon, rectal, breast, and prostate cancers. Lycopene is a powerful antioxidant that acts against cancerous cell formation. Free radicals in the body can be reduced by lycopene which lowers the risk of heart disease, age related disease in eyes, and diabetes. Lycopene prevents skin damage from UV rays and protects the skin. Vitamin C is a powerful antioxidant that boosts the immune system and protects the body from diseases.

Lutein and zeaxanthin protect the eyes from the age related macular defects in elderly people by filtering harmful UV rays.

Potassium in tomatoes helps control heart rate and blood pressure.

Studies have shown that type 1 diabetics who consume high-fibre diets have lower blood glucose levels and type 2 diabetics may have improved blood sugar, lipids and insulin levels.

Tomatoes contain high water content and fibre that can help to keep you hydrated and your bowel movements regular. Fibre is essential for minimizing constipation and adding bulk to the stool.

In pregnancy folic acid intake is essential for pregnant women to protect against neural tube defects in infants. The folic acid found in tomatoes may also help with depression by preventing an excess of homocysteine from forming in the body, which can prevent blood and other nutrients from reaching the brain. Excess homocysteine interferes with the production of the feel-good hormones serotonin, dopamine, and norepinephrine, which regulate not only mood, but sleep and appetite as well.

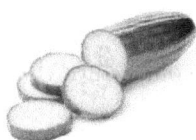

CUCUMBER

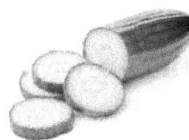

NUTRITION FACTS

VITAMINS – Vitamin C (2.8mg), Thiamin (0.027mg), Riboflavin (0.033mg), Niacin (0.098mg), Vitamin B6 (0.04mg), Folate (7µg), Vitamin A (5µg), Vitamin E (0.03mg), and Vitamin K (16.4µg)

MINERALS – Calcium (16mg), Iron (0.28mg), Magnesium (13mg), Phosphorus (24mg), Potassium (147mg), Sodium (2mg) and Zinc (0.2mg).

[USDA national nutrient database, 2015]

Nutrient	Value per 100g
Energy	15kcal
Protein	0.65g
Fat	0.11g
Carbohydrate	3.63g
Fibre	0.5g
Sugar	1.67g

HEALTH BENEFITS

☆ **Cardiovascular benefits**

☆ **Hydration**

☆ **Anti-aging**

☆ **Anti-inflammatory benefits**

☆ **Regulates blood sugar and glucose levels**

The high water content of this vegetable promotes urination and prevents kidney stones, and provides cooling effect in the body. During the hot summer months cucumbers helps to prevent dehydration. The good source of fibre in cucumbers helps in easy digestion. This vegetable can be used topically to relieve skin afflictions like sun burns and puffy eyes. Silica and antioxidants help to rejuvenate the skin.

When used topically, cucumber has a cooling and soothing effect that decreases swelling, irritation and inflammation. Cucumber slices can be placed on the eyes to decrease morning puffiness or placed on the skin to alleviate and treat sunburn.

Cucumbers are a good source of potassium which is a component of body fluid and maintains the sodium level in the blood, which reduces blood pressure.

Vitamin A and C, and beta carotene are antioxidants that reduce the effect of free radical damage in the body.

Cucumbers contain sterols which help to lower cholesterol levels in the blood.

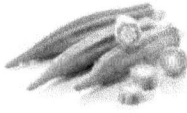

OKRA

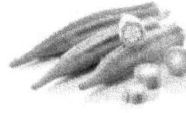

NUTRITION FACTS

VITAMINS – Vitamin C (23mg), Thiamin (0.2mg), Riboflavin (0.06mg), Niacin (1mg), Vitamin B6 (0.215mg), Folate (60μg), Vitamin A (36μg), Vitamin E (0.27mg), and Vitamin K (31.3μg)

MINERALS – Calcium (82mg), Iron (0.62mg), Magnesium (57mg), Phosphorus (61mg), Potassium (299mg), Sodium (7mg) and Zinc (0.58mg).

[USDA national nutrient database, 2015]

Nutrient	Value per 100g
Energy	33kcal
Protein	1.93g
Fat	0.19g
Carbohydrate	7.45g
Fibre	3.2g
Sugar	1.48g

HEALTH BENEFITS

☆ **Prevents constipation and promotes easy bowel movements**

☆ **Helps control cholesterol**

☆ **Antioxidant properties which are essential for vision**

☆ **Anti-cancer**

☆ **Helps strengthen bones**

☆ **Helps develop good immunity**

☆ **Decreases incidences of neural tube defects**

Okra is also known as 'lady's fingers'. Okra is rich in vitamins, minerals, fibre and antioxidants. The high fibre and mucilaginous content in okra helps in easy digestion; the soluble fibre in okra, called pectin, absorbs water and helps in peristalsis movement in the colon and relieves constipation.

The fibre in okra helps to reduce blood sugar by slowing down the sugar absorption in the blood.

Vitamin A is good for healthy mucus membranes and skin. Vitamin C helps the body develop immunity against infectious agents and reduces harmful free radicals. Folic acid in okra is good for nerve health.

Okra are composed of healthy amounts of vitamin A, and flavonoid anti-oxidants such as beta-carotene, xanthin and lutein. It is one of the vegetables with highest levels of these anti-oxidants. These compounds are known to have antioxidant properties and are essential for vision.

They are also rich in B-complex group of vitamins like niacin, vitamin B6 (pyridoxine), thiamin and pantothenic acid. The pods also contain good amounts of vitamin K. Vitamin K is a co-factor for blood clotting enzymes and is required for strengthening of bones.

Fresh okra are a good source of folates. Consumption of foods rich in folate, especially during the pre-conception period helps decrease the incidence of neural tube defects in the offspring.

Okra being rich in flavonoids helps to protect from lung and oral cavity cancers.

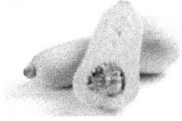

BUTTERNUT SQUASH

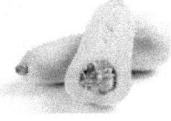

NUTRITION FACTS

VITAMINS – Vitamin C (21mg), Thiamin (0.1mg), Riboflavin (0.02mg), Niacin (1.2mg), Vitamin B6 (0.154mg), Folate (27µg), Vitamin A (532µg), Vitamin E (1.44mg), and Vitamin K (1.1µg)

MINERALS – Calcium (48mg), Iron (0.7mg), Magnesium (34mg), Phosphorus (33mg), Potassium (352mg), Sodium (4mg) and Zinc (0.15mg).

[USDA national nutrient database, 2015]

Nutrient	Value per 100g
Energy	45kcal
Protein	1g
Fat	0.1g
Carbohydrate	11.69g
Fibre	2g
Sugar	2.2g

HEALTH BENEFITS

☆ **Lowering and preventing high blood pressure**

☆ **Preventing asthma**

☆ **Lowering the risk of cancers**

☆ **Managing diabetes**

☆ **Healthy looking skin and hair**

☆ **Prevents constipation and promotes easy bowel movements**

☆ **Boosting immune function**

☆ **Antioxidant benefits**

Butternut squash is rich in dietary fibre, vitamin A, folate, and antioxidants. Vitamin A is a powerful antioxidant that is good for maintaining the skin and mucous membranes. It is also essential for good vision. Vitamin A protects the body against lung cancer and oral cavity cancer.

Recent research has found that butternut squash has antioxidants that help in the prevention of prostate cancer, colon cancer and breast cancer.

Vitamin C helps to make collagen, which is a major component of cartilage which aids in joint support and flexibility. It is rich in carotene, lutein-zeaxanthin, and criptoxanthin, which are all powerful antioxidants that protect the body from free radicals. The seeds of this squash contain omega-6-fatty acids and oleic acid which are good for heart and brain health.

The high potassium content in butternut squash helps to maintain a healthy blood pressure.

Also the risk of developing asthma are reduced in people who consume a high amount of beta-carotene, the antioxidant that gives butternut squash their bright orange pigments.

Type 1 diabetics who consume high-fibre diets have lower overall blood sugar levels, while type 2 diabetics have improved blood sugar, lipids and insulin levels.

Butternut squash is also great for your skin as it contains a high content of vitamin A, which is needed for sebum production that keeps hair moisturized. Vitamin A plays an important role in the growth of all bodily tissues, including skin and hair.

The high fibre content helps to prevent constipation and promote a healthy digestive tract.

Plant foods like butternut squash that are high in both vitamin C and beta-carotene offer an immunity boost from their powerful combination of nutrients. Some studies have shown that high-fibre foods may also offer improved immune function.

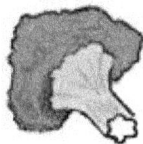

BROCCOLI

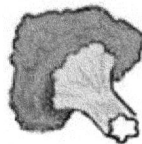

NUTRITION FACTS

VITAMINS – Vitamin C (89.2mg),
Thiamin (0.071mg), Riboflavin (0.117mg),
Niacin (0.639mg), Vitamin B6 (0.175mg),
Folate (63μg), Vitamin A (31μg),
Vitamin E (0.78mg), and
Vitamin K (101.6μg)

MINERALS – Calcium (47mg),
Iron (0.73mg), Magnesium (21mg),
Phosphorus (66mg), Potassium (316mg),
Sodium (33mg) and Zinc (0.41mg).

[USDA national nutrient database, 2015]

Nutrient	Value per 100g
Energy	34kcal
Protein	2.82g
Fat	0.37g
Carbohydrate	6.64g
Fibre	2.6g
Sugar	1.7g

HEALTH BENEFITS

☆ **Fights against cancer**

☆ **Anti-aging**

☆ **Improves bone health**

☆ **Protection from chronic disease**

☆ **Prevent constipations and promotes easy bowel movements**

Broccolis contain sulforaphane, the sulfur-containing compound that gives cruciferous bitter bite, studies have suggested that this is what gives them their cancer-fighting power.

An important vitamin that broccoli contains is folate, which has shown to decrease the risk of breast cancer in women. Adequate intake of dietary folate (in food) has also shown promising results in protecting against colon, stomach, pancreatic and cervical cancers.

Poor vitamin K intake is linked with a high risk of bone fracture. The high content of vitamin K in broccoli helps to improve bone health by improving calcium absorption and reducing urinary excretion of calcium.

The antioxidant vitamin C, when eaten in its natural form (in fresh produce as opposed to supplement form) can help to fight skin damage caused by the sun and pollution, reduce wrinkles and improve overall skin texture.

Eating foods with a natural fibre content like broccoli can prevent constipation and promotes easy bowel movement. Studies have shown that fibre may also play a role in regulating the immune system and inflammation.

High fibre intakes has been shown to be associated with lowering the risks of developing coronary heart disease, stroke, hypertension, diabetes, obesity, and certain gastrointestinal diseases.

Increased fibre intake has also been shown to lower blood pressure and cholesterol levels and improve insulin sensitivity.

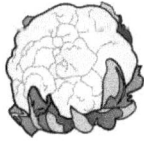

CAULIFLOWER

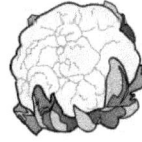

NUTRITION FACTS

VITAMINS – Vitamin C (48.2mg), Thiamin (0.05mg), Riboflavin (0.06mg), Niacin (0.507mg), Vitamin B6 (0.184mg), Folate (57µg), Vitamin E (0.08mg), and Vitamin K (15.5µg)

MINERALS – Calcium (22mg), Iron (0.42mg), Magnesium (15mg), Phosphorus (44mg), Potassium (299mg), Sodium (30mg) and Zinc (0.27mg).

[USDA national nutrient database, 2015]

Nutrient	Value per 100g
Energy	25kcal
Protein	1.92g
Fat	0.28g
Carbohydrate	4.97g
Fibre	2g
Sugar	1.91g

HEALTH BENEFITS

☆ **Anti-cancer**

☆ **Prevents constipation and promotes easy bowel movements**

☆ **Cognitive benefits**

☆ **Promotes strong bones**

Cauliflower contains antioxidants that help prevent cellular mutations and reduce oxidative stress from free radicals. One of these is indole-3-carbinol or I3C, which has been shown to reduce the risk of breast and reproductive cancers in men and women. Recent studies have shown that sulfur-containing compounds (namely sulforaphane) that give cruciferous vegetables their bitter bite are also what give them their cancer-fighting power.

The high fibre and water content found in cauliflower, helps to prevent constipation, maintain a healthy digestive tract and lower the risk of colon cancer.

Recent studies have shown that dietary fibre may play a role in regulating the immune system and inflammation, consequently decreasing the risk of inflammation-related conditions such as cardiovascular disease, diabetes, cancer, and obesity.

Choline is a very important and versatile "vitamin-like factor" in cauliflower that helps with sleep, muscle movement, learning and memory. Choline also helps to maintain the structure of cellular membranes, aids in the transmission of nerve impulses, assists in the absorption of fat and reduces chronic inflammation.

Low intakes of vitamin K have been associated with a higher risk for bone fracture and osteoporosis. Adequate vitamin K consumption improves bone health by acting as a modifier of bone matrix proteins, improving calcium absorption and reducing urinary excretion of calcium.

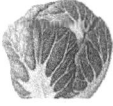

BRUSSELS SPROUTS

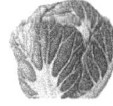

NUTRITION FACTS

VITAMINS – Vitamin C (85mg),
Thiamin (0.139mg), Riboflavin (0.09mg),
Niacin (0.745mg), Vitamin B6 (0.219mg),
Folate (61µg), Vitamin A (38µg),
Vitamin E (0.88mg), and Vitamin K (177µg)

MINERALS – Calcium (42mg),
Iron (1.4mg), Magnesium (23mg),
Phosphorus (69mg), Potassium (389mg),
Sodium (25mg) and Zinc (0.42mg).

[USDA national nutrient database, 2015]

Nutrient	Value per 100g
Energy	43kcal
Protein	3.38g
Fat	0.3g
Carbohydrate	8.95g
Fibre	3.8g
Sugar	2.2g

HEALTH BENEFITS

☆ **Anti-cancer**

☆ **Anti-aging**

☆ **Improves bone health**

☆ **Helps manage diabetes**

☆ **Prevents macular degeneration**

☆ **Healthy eyes**

Intake of high amounts of cruciferous vegetables like brussels sprouts
has been associated with a lower risk of cancer. The sulfur-containing
compounds (namely sulforaphane) that found in brussels sprouts that
give them their bitter bite are also what give them their cancer-fighting
power.

Brussels sprouts also contain a high amount of chlorophyll, which can block the carcinogenic effects of heterocyclic amines generated when grilling meats at a high temperature. If you tend to like your grilled foods charred, make sure to pair them with green vegetables to decrease your risk.

Low intakes of vitamin K have been associated with a higher risk for bone fracture. Adequate vitamin K consumption improves bone health by acting as a modifier of bone matrix proteins, improving calcium absorption and reducing urinary excretion of calcium.

Many green vegetables contain an antioxidant known as alpha-lipoic acid that has been shown to lower glucose levels, increase insulin sensitivity and prevent oxidative stress-induced changes in patients with diabetes. Studies on alpha-lipoic acid have also shown decreases in peripheral neuropathy or autonomic neuropathy in diabetics.

Making sure you get your daily requirement of vitamin C has been shown to help keep eyes healthy by providing increased protection against UV light damage.

Eating just one serving of brussels sprouts per day would ensure you are getting enough of this important nutrient. Another antioxidant in brussels sprouts, zeaxanthin, filters out harmful blue light rays and is thought to play a protective role in eye health and possibly ward off damage from macular degeneration.

The antioxidant vitamin C, when eaten in its natural form (in fresh produce as opposed to supplement form) or applied topically, can help to fight skin damage caused by the sun and pollution, reduce wrinkles and improve overall skin texture. Vitamin C plays a vital role in the formation of collagen, the main support system of skin.

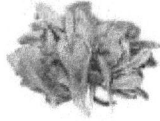

KALE

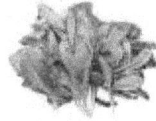

NUTRITION FACTS

VITAMINS – Vitamin C (120mg), Thiamin (0.11mg), Riboflavin (0.13mg), Niacin (1mg), Vitamin B6 (0.271mg), Folate (141µg), Vitamin A (500µg), Vitamin E (1.54mg), and Vitamin K (704.8µg)

MINERALS – Calcium (150mg), Iron (1.47mg), Magnesium (47mg), Phosphorus (92mg), Potassium (491mg), Sodium (38mg) and Zinc (0.56mg).

[USDA national nutrient database, 2015]

Nutrient	Value per 100g
Energy	49kcal
Protein	4.28g
Fat	0.93g
Carbohydrate	8.75g
Fibre	3.6g
Sugar	2.26g

HEALTH BENEFITS

☆ **Anti-cancer**

☆ **Bone health**

☆ **Prevents constipation and easy bowel movements**

☆ **Healthier skin and hair**

☆ **Beneficial for diabetics**

☆ **Cardiovascular benefits**

☆ **Antioxidant benefits**

The high fibre content in kale help type 1 diabetics have lower blood glucose levels and may help improve blood sugar, lipids and insulin levels in type 2 diabetics. Kale also contains an antioxidant known as alpha-lipoic acid, which has been shown to lower glucose levels, increase insulin sensitivity and prevent oxidative stress-induced changes in patients with diabetes.

Kale is packed with nutrition making it one of the healthiest foods available.

The fibre, potassium, vitamin C and B6 content in kale all help provide cardiovascular benefits. An increase in potassium intake along with a decrease in sodium intake is the most important dietary change that a person can make to reduce their risk of cardiovascular disease.

Risk of stroke can be reduced due to the high potassium content, as well as protection against loss of muscle mass, preservation of bone mineral density and reduction in the formation of kidney stones.

It is known that increased intake of potassium and reduced intake of sodium is also associated with decreasing blood pressure levels due to potassium's vasodilation effects.

Kale and other green vegetables that contain chlorophyll have been shown to be effective at blocking the carcinogenic effects of heterocyclic amines, which are generated when grilling foods at a high temperature. If you tend to like your grilled foods charred, make sure to pair them with green vegetables to help negate these effects.

Low intakes of vitamin K have been associated with a higher risk for bone fracture. Adequate vitamin K consumption is important for good health, as it acts as a modifier of bone matrix proteins, improves calcium absorption and may reduce urinary excretion of calcium.

Kale is high in fibre and water content, both of which help to prevent constipation and promote regularity and a healthy digestive tract.

Kale is high in vitamin A, a nutrient required for sebum production to keep hair moisturized. Vitamin A is also necessary for the growth of all bodily tissues, including skin and hair.

Adequate intake of vitamin C, which kale can provide, is needed for the building and maintenance of collagen, which provides structure to skin and hair.

Iron-deficiency is a common cause of hair loss, which can be prevented by an adequate intake of iron-rich foods, like kale.

"FOR A HEALTHY BODY FOR YOU AND ME, HEALTHY EATING IS THE KEY"

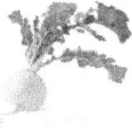

TURNIPS

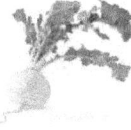

NUTRITION FACTS

VITAMINS – Vitamin C (21mg), Thiamin (0.04mg), Riboflavin (0.03mg), Niacin (0.4mg), Vitamin B6 (0.09mg), Folate (15µg), Vitamin E (0.03mg), and Vitamin K (0.1µg)

MINERALS – Calcium (30mg), Iron (0.3mg), Magnesium (11mg), Phosphorus (27mg), Potassium (191mg), Sodium (67mg) and Zinc (0.27mg).

[USDA national nutrient database, 2015]

Nutrient	Value per 100g
Energy	28kcal
Protein	0.9g
Fat	0.1g
Carbohydrate	6.43g
Fibre	1.8g
Sugar	3.8g

HEALTH BENEFITS

☆ **Anti-cancer**

☆ **Treating diverticulitis**

☆ **Lowers blood pressure**

☆ **Healthier vision**

☆ **Prevents constipation and promotes easy bowel movements**

The high fibre content in turnips have been shown to decrease the prevalence in flare-ups of diverticulitis by absorbing water in the colon and making bowel movements easier to pass.

Foods containing dietary nitrates like turnips have been shown to have multiple vascular benefits, including lowering blood pressure, inhibiting platelet aggregation, and preserving or improving endothelial dysfunction.

Turnips also have potassium, which is thought to bring blood pressure down by releasing sodium out of the body and helping arteries dilate.

Sulforaphane compound found in turnips are what gives the vegetable the bitter taste and this is what gives them their cancer-fighting power as well. It has the ability to delay or impede cancer such as melanoma, esophageal, prostate and pancreatic cancers.

The fibre content in turnips also prevents constipation and promotes regularity for a healthy digestive tract.

Recent studies have shown that the fibre content plays a key role the immune system and inflammation, consequently decreasing the risk of inflammation-related conditions such as cardiovascular disease, diabetes, cancer and obesity.

Turnips also contain an adequate content of vitamin C which has shown to help keep eyes healthy by providing increased protection against UV light damage.

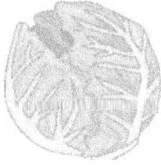

CABBAGE

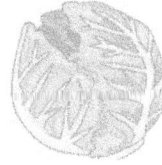

NUTRITION FACTS

VITAMINS – Vitamin C (36.6mg),
Thiamin (0.061mg), Riboflavin (0.04mg),
Niacin (0.234mg), Vitamin B6 (0.124mg),
Folate (43µg), Vitamin A (5µg),
Vitamin E (0.15mg), and Vitamin K (76µg)

MINERALS – Calcium (40mg),
Iron (0.47mg), Magnesium (12mg),
Phosphorus (26mg), Potassium (170mg),
Sodium (18mg) and Zinc (0.18mg).

[USDA national nutrient database, 2015]

Nutrient	Value per 100g
Energy	25kcal
Protein	1.28g
Fat	0.1g
Carbohydrate	5.8g
Fibre	2.5g
Sugar	3.2g

HEALTH BENEFITS

☆ **Anti-cancer**

☆ **Cardiovascular benefits**

☆ **Healthier immune and digestive systems**

☆ **Prevents constipation**

Sulforaphane is also found in cabbage which helps lowers the risk of cancer such as melanoma, esophageal, prostate and pancreatic cancers. The sulphur compounds is what gives cruciferous vegetables their bitter taste.

Studies have shown that sulforaphane has the power to inhibit the harmful enzyme histone deacetylase (HDAC), known to be involved in the progression of cancer cells. The ability to stop HDAC enzymes could make sulforaphane-containing foods a potentially powerful part of cancer treatment.

Studies conducted at the University of Missouri have shown that apigenin, another natural chemical found in cabbage, helps decrease the size of tumours in an aggressive form of breast cancer. Thus has the has potential to be used as a non-toxic treatment for cancer in the future.

Studies have shown that the intake of flavonoid-rich foods have been related to a lower risk from cardiovascular diseases. The high polyphenol content present in cabbages help prevent platelet build-up and is beneficial in reducing blood pressure.

The fibre and water content in cabbage also helps to prevent constipation and maintain a healthy digestive tract. Eating adequate fibre promotes regularity, which is crucial for the daily excretion toxins through the bile and stool.

Recent studies have shown that dietary fibre may even play a role in regulating the immune system and inflammation, consequently decreasing the risk of inflammation-related conditions such as cardiovascular disease, diabetes, cancer and obesity.

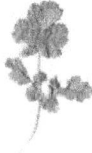

WATERCRESS

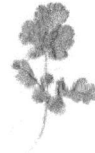

NUTRITION FACTS

VITAMINS – Vitamin C (43mg), Thiamin (0.09mg), Riboflavin (0.12mg), Niacin (0.2mg), Vitamin B6 (0.129mg), Folate (9μg), Vitamin A (160μg), Vitamin E (1mg), and Vitamin K (250μg)

MINERALS – Calcium (120mg), Iron (0.2mg), Magnesium (21mg), Phosphorus (60mg), Potassium (330mg), Sodium (41mg) and Zinc (0.11mg).

[USDA national nutrient database, 2015]

Nutrient	Value per 100g
Energy	11kcal
Protein	2.3g
Fat	0.1g
Carbohydrate	1.29g
Fibre	0.5g
Sugar	0.2g

HEALTH BENEFITS

☆ **Anti-cancer**

☆ **Cardiovascular benefits**

☆ **Healthier bones**

☆ **Beneficial for diabetics**

Watercress is also one of the cruciferous vegetables that has been known to be associated with lowering the risk of lung and colon cancer. It is the sulfur-containing compounds (namely sulforaphane) that give the vegetable its bitter taste and its cancer-fighting power.

The high amounts of chlorophyll present in watercress has shown to be effective at blocking the carcinogenic effects of heterocyclic amines generated when grilling foods at a high temperature.

Watercress contain all three minerals, calcium, magnesium and potassium, which have thought to bring down blood pressure by releasing sodium out of the body and helping arteries dilate as well as helping to improve intake.

Dietary nitrates present in watercress have been shown to have multiple vascular benefits, including reducing blood pressure, inhibiting platelet aggregation, and preserving or improving endothelial dysfunction.

Consumption of watercress improves bone health by acting as a modifier of bone matrix proteins, improving calcium absorption and reducing urinary excretion of calcium, all due to the higher levels of vitamin K found in watercress.

Watercress helps lower glucose levels as it contains the antioxidant alpha-lipoic acid and increases insulin sensitivity and prevents oxidative stress-induced changes in patients with diabetes. Research has shown decreases in peripheral neuropathy or autonomic neuropathy in diabetics.

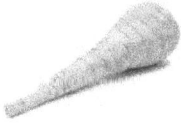

PARSNIPS

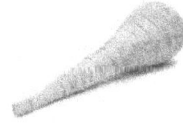

NUTRITION FACTS

VITAMINS – Vitamin C (17mg), Thiamin (0.09mg), Riboflavin (0.05mg), Niacin (0.7mg), Vitamin B6 (0.09mg), Folate (67μg), Vitamin E (1.49mg), and Vitamin K (22.5μg)

MINERALS – Calcium (36mg), Iron (0.59mg), Magnesium (29mg), Phosphorus (71mg), Potassium (375mg), Sodium (10mg) and Zinc (0.59mg).

[USDA national nutrient database, 2015]

Nutrient	Value per 100g
Energy	75kcal
Protein	1.2g
Fat	0.3g
Carbohydrate	17.99g
Fibre	4.9g
Sugar	4.8g

HEALTH BENEFITS

☆ **Anti-cancer**

☆ **Cardiovascular benefits**

☆ **Anti-inflammatory benefits**

☆ **Prevents constipation**

☆ **Reduce cholesterol**

☆ **Healthier teeth and gums**

Even though parsnips contain more sugar than carrots, radish and turnips its sweet, juicy root is rich in several health-benefiting phytonutrients, vitamins, minerals, and fibres.

Parsnips are an excellent sources of soluble and insoluble dietary fibres. The content of fibre present helps to reduce blood cholesterol levels, and helps prevent constipation.

Antioxidants such as falcarinol, falcarindiol, panaxydiol, and methyl-falcarindiol are also present parsnips. These compounds have been shown to cause anti-inflammatory, anti-fungal, and anti-cancer functions and offer protection from colon cancer and acute lymphoblastic leukemia (ALL).

Vitamin C present in the fresh roots of parsnips is a powerful water-soluble anti-oxidant. It helps the human body maintain healthy connective tissue, teeth, and gum. Its anti-oxidant property helps protect from diseases and cancers by scavenging harmful free radicals from the body.

The roots are also rich in folic acid, vitamin B6, thiamin, vitamin K and vitamin E.

In addition, it also has healthy levels of minerals like iron, calcium, copper, potassium, manganese and phosphorus. Potassium is an important component of cell and body fluids that helps control heart rate and blood pressure by the countering effects of sodium.

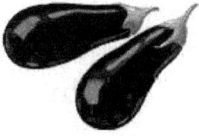

AUBERGINE

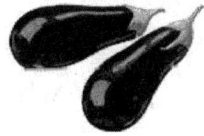

NUTRITION FACTS

VITAMINS – Vitamin C (2.2mg), Thiamin (0.039mg), Riboflavin (0.037mg), Niacin (0.649mg), Vitamin B6 (0.084mg), Folate (22µg), Vitamin A (1µg), Vitamin E (0.3mg), and Vitamin K (3.5µg)

MINERALS – Calcium (9mg), Iron (0.23mg), Magnesium (14mg), Phosphorus (24mg), Potassium (229mg), Sodium (2mg) and Zinc (0.16mg).

[USDA national nutrient database, 2015]

Nutrient	Value per 100g
Energy	25kcal
Protein	0.98g
Fat	0.18g
Carbohydrate	5.88g
Fibre	3g
Sugar	3.53g

HEALTH BENEFITS

☆ **Anti-cancer**

☆ **Cardiovascular benefits**

☆ **Lowers blood cholesterol**

☆ **Antioxidant benefits**

The phytonutrient, fibre, potassium, vitamin C, vitamin B6 content present in aubergines, also known as eggplants, all contribute to a healthier cardiovascular system. Research have shown that the consumption of foods containing even small quantities of flavonoids is affiliated with a lower risk of mortality from heart disease as well as the reduction of blood pressure, especially the flavonoids known as anthocyanins.

Research has shown that the consumption of aubergines can help reduce blood cholesterol as well as a significant decrease in weight.

It has been found that aubergines contain a significant amount of chlorogenic acid, which is one of the most powerful free radical scavengers found in plants. Chlorogenic acid has been shown to decrease LDL (low density lipids) levels, and also serves as an antimicrobial, antiviral, and anticarcinogenic agent.

Aubergines also contain polyphenols which have been found to exhibit anti-cancer effects. Anthocyanins and chlorogenic acid function as antioxidants and anti-inflammatory compounds. They protect body cells from damage caused by free radicals and in turn prevent tumour growth and invasion and spread of cancer cells. They also stimulate detoxifying enzymes within cells and promote death of cancer cells.

Studies undertaken on animals have shown that nasunin, an anthocyaninpresent in the skin of aubergines, is a powerful antioxidant that protects the lipids comprising cell membranes in brain cells from free radical damage. It has also been proven to help facilitate the transport of nutrients into the cell and wastes out.

Research has shown inhibition of neuro-inflammation and blood flow to the brain can be facilitated by anthocyanins found in aubergines. This helps prevent age-related mental disorders and also improves memory.

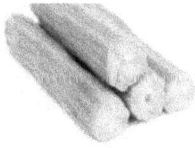

DRUMSTICK

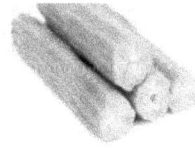

NUTRITION FACTS

VITAMINS – Vitamin C (141mg), Thiamin (0.053mg), Riboflavin (0.074mg), Niacin (0.62mg), Vitamin B6 (0.12mg), Folate (44μg) and Vitamin A (4μg)

MINERALS – Calcium (30mg), Iron (0.36mg), Magnesium (45mg), Phosphorus (50mg), Potassium (461mg), Sodium (42mg) and Zinc (0.45mg).

[USDA national nutrient database, 2015]

Nutrient	Value per 100g
Energy	37kcal
Protein	2.1g
Fat	0.2g
Carbohydrate	8.53g
Fibre	3.2g

HEALTH BENEFITS

☆ **Anti-cancer**

☆ **Cardiovascular benefits**

☆ **Lowers blood cholesterol**

☆ **Antioxidant benefits**

☆ **Healthier skin**

☆ **Beneficial both pre and post pregnancy**

☆ **Beneficial during colds and sore throats**

☆ **Helps ease asthma and lung problems**

Moringa oleifera is the scientific name for what is known popularly as drumstick tree, is a tropical plant grown for its nutritious leafy-greens, flower buds, and mineral-rich green fruit pods. This plant is thought to be originated in the sub-Himalayan forests of the Indian subcontinent. It possesses horseradish-like root and, hence, known to the western world as horseradish tree. Their young, tender seed pods are popularly known as 'murnga' in Tamil, and 'malunggay' in the Philippines.

The fresh pods and seeds of a drumstick are a good source of oleic acid, a health-benefiting monounsaturated fat.

Fresh drumstick pods are an excellent source of vitamin C which helps the body develop immunity against infectious agents, and scavenge harmful oxygen-free radicals from the body.

Moringa also contains many vital vitamins such as folates, vitamin B6, thiamin, riboflavin, pantothenic acid, and niacin.

Furthermore, it consists of minerals like calcium, iron, copper, manganese, zinc, selenium, and magnesium. Iron helps alleviate anaemia. Calcium is required for bone mineralisation. Zinc plays a vital role in hair-growth, spermatogenesis, and skin health.

Drumsticks are said to be a great blood purifiers. It is also recommended to pregnant women as it helps ease any kind of pre and post-delivery complications. It also has been considered to help increase breast milk production in the early period after childbirth.

Drumsticks have also been known to ease chest congestions, coughs and sore throats. Inhaling steam of water in which drumsticks have been boiled helps ease asthma and other lung problem.

Finally consumption of drumstick juice greatly has been known to add a glow on one's face. Thus gives a healthier looking skin complexion.

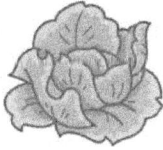

LETTUCE

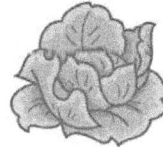

NUTRITION FACTS

VITAMINS – Vitamin C (9.2mg), Thiamin (0.07mg), Riboflavin (0.08mg), Niacin (0.375mg), Vitamin B6 (0.09mg), Folate (38µg), Vitamin A (370µg), Vitamin E (0.22mg) and Vitamin K (126.3µg)

MINERALS – Calcium (36mg), Iron (0.86mg), Magnesium (13mg), Phosphorus (29mg), Potassium (194mg), Sodium (28mg) and Zinc (0.18mg).

[USDA national nutrient database, 2015]

Nutrient	Value per 100g
Energy	15kcal
Protein	1.36g
Fat	0.15g
Carbohydrate	2.87g
Fibre	1.3g
Sugar	0.78g

HEALTH BENEFITS

☆ **Anti-cancer**

☆ **Cardiovascular benefits**

☆ **Antioxidant benefits**

☆ **Protects against Alzheimer's disease and osteoporosis**

☆ **Healthier skin**

☆ **Prevents tube defects in baby (foetus) during pregnancy**

☆ **Beneficial during colds and sore throats**

☆ **Helps ease asthma and lung problems**

Lettuce contains many phytonutrients that possess health promoting and disease prevention properties.

Lettuce is an excellent source of vitamin A and beta carotenes. These compounds have antioxidant properties. Vitamin A is required for maintaining healthy mucus membranes and skin, and is also essential for vision. Consumption of natural fruits and vegetables rich in flavonoids helps to protect the body from lung and oral cavity cancers.

It is a rich source of vitamin K. Vitamin K has a potential role in the bone metabolism where it thought to increase bone mass by promoting osteotrophic activity inside the bone cells. It also has established role in Alzheimer's disease patients by limiting neuronal damage in the brain.

Fresh leaves contain good amounts folates and vitamin C. Folates are part of co-factors in the enzyme metabolism required for DNA synthesis and therefore, play a vital role in prevention of the neural tube defects in the baby (fetus) during pregnancy.

Vitamin C is a powerful natural antioxidant; regular consumption of foods rich in vitamin C helps the body develop resistance against infectious agents and scavenge harmful, pro-inflammatory free radicals.

Zeaxanthin, an important dietary carotenoid in lettuce, is selectively absorbed into the retinal macula lutea, where it thought to provide antioxidant and filter UV rays falling on the retina. Diet rich in xanthin and carotenes is thought to offer some protection against age-related macular disease (ARMD) in the elderly.

It also contains good amounts of minerals like iron, calcium, magnesium, and potassium, which are very essential for body metabolism. Potassium is an important component of cell and body fluids that helps controlling heart rate and blood pressure. Manganese is used by the body as a co-factor for the antioxidant enzyme, superoxide dismutase. Copper is required in the production of red blood cells. Iron is essential for red blood cell formation.

It is rich in B-complex group of vitamins like thiamin, vitamin B6 (pyridoxine) and riboflavins.

Regular inclusion of lettuce in salads is known to prevent osteoporosis, iron-deficiency anaemia, and believed to protect from cardiovascular diseases, ARMD, Alzheimer's disease and cancers.

"WITH BROCCOLI AND KALE YOU CAN'T FAIL"

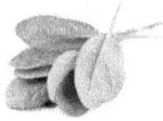

SPINACH

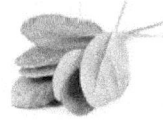

NUTRITION FACTS

VITAMINS – Vitamin C (28.1mg), Thiamin (0.078mg), Riboflavin (0.189mg), Niacin (0.724mg), Vitamin B6 (0.195mg), Folate (194µg), Vitamin A (469µg), Vitamin E (2.03mg) and Vitamin K (482.9µg)

MINERALS – Calcium (99mg), Iron (2.71mg), Magnesium (79mg), Phosphorus (49mg), Potassium (558mg), Sodium (79mg) and Zinc (0.53mg).

[USDA national nutrient database, 2015]

Nutrient	Value per 100g
Energy	23kcal
Protein	2.86g
Fat	0.39g
Carbohydrate	3.63g
Fibre	2.2g
Sugar	0.42g

HEALTH BENEFITS

☆ **Helps manage diabetes**

☆ **Antioxidant benefits**

☆ **Anti-cancer**

☆ **Cardiovascular benefits**

☆ **Antioxidant benefits**

☆ **Anti-asthma**

☆ **Lowers blood pressure**

☆ **Helps prevent constipation**

☆ **Healthier skin and hair**

Spinach contains an antioxidant known as alpha-lipoic acid, which has been shown to lower glucose levels, increase insulin sensitivity and prevent oxidative stress-induced changes in patients with diabetes.

Chlorophyll present in spinach has shown to be effective at blocking the carcinogenic effects of heterocyclic amines which are generated when grilling foods at a high temperature thus helping to prevent cancer.

Consumption of spinach lowers the risk of developing asthma due to the nutrients known as beta-carotene of which spinach is an excellent source.

Due to the high potassium content, spinach is recommended to those with high blood pressure to negate the effects of sodium in the body. A low potassium intake may be just as big of a risk factor in developing

Spinach is high in fibre and water content, both of which help to prevent constipation and promote a healthy digestive tract.

The high source of vitamin A in spinach helps to keep the hair moisturized. Vitamin A is also necessary for the growth of all bodily tissues, including skin and hair. Spinach and other leafy greens high in vitamin C helps provide structure to skin and hair.

Iron-deficiency is known to be a common cause of hair loss. This can be prevented by an adequate intake of iron-rich foods, like spinach.

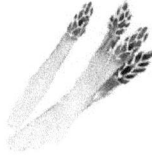

ASPARAGUS

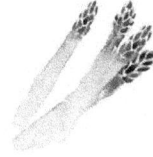

NUTRITION FACTS

VITAMINS – Vitamin C (5.6mg),
Thiamin (0.143mg), Riboflavin (0.141mg),
Niacin (0.978mg), Vitamin B6 (0.091mg),
Folate (52µg), Vitamin A (38µg),
Vitamin E (1.13mg) and Vitamin K (41.6µg)

MINERALS – Calcium (24mg),
Iron (2.14mg), Magnesium (14mg),
Phosphorus (52mg), Potassium (202mg),
Sodium (2mg) and Zinc (0.54mg).

[USDA national nutrient database, 2015]

Nutrient	Value per 100g
Energy	20kcal
Protein	2.2g
Fat	0.12g
Carbohydrate	3.88g
Fibre	2.1g
Sugar	1.88g

HEALTH BENEFITS

☆ **Decreased risk of birth defects**

☆ **Lowered risk of depression**

☆ **Cardiovascular benefits**

☆ **Prevention of osteoporosis**

☆ **Anti-cancer**

Asparagus has been known to decrease the risk of obesity, diabetes, heart disease and overall mortality while promoting a healthy complexion and hair, increased energy and overall lower weight.

Asparagus is extremely important during periods of rapid growth such as pregnancy, infancy and adolescence due to its best natural source of folate.

Folic acid is essential for pregnant women to protect their infants against miscarriage and neural tube defects. Recent studies have shown that folate is just as much essential.

Folate may help ward off depression by preventing an excess of homocysteine from forming in the body, which can block blood and other nutrients from reaching the brain. Excess homocysteine interferes with the production of the feel-good hormones serotonin, dopamine, and norepinephrine, which regulate not only mood, but sleep and appetite as well.

Low levels of folate intake have been shown to increase the risk of breast cancer in women. Adequate intake of dietary folate (in food) has also shown promise in protecting against colon, stomach, pancreatic and cervical cancers.

Asparagus consists of high levels of vitamin K which is essential to improve bone health by improving calcium absorption and reducing urinary excretion of calcium. The iron in asparagus also plays a crucial role in maintaining the strength

The high fibre and water content both help to prevent constipation, maintain a healthy lifestyle

Asparagus is high in both fibre and water content, which helps to prevent constipation, maintain a healthy digestive tract and lower the risk of colon cancer.

Adequate fibre promotes regularity, which is crucial for the daily excretion of toxins through the bile and stool. Recent studies have shown that dietary fibre may also play a role in regulating the immune system and inflammation, consequently decreasing the risk of inflammation-related conditions such as cardiovascular disease, diabetes, cancer and obesity.

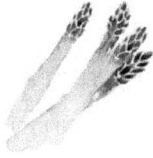

LEEKS

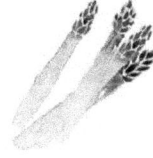

NUTRITION FACTS

VITAMINS – Vitamin C (12mg),
Thiamin (0.06mg), Riboflavin (0.03mg),
Niacin (0.4mg), Vitamin B6 (0.233mg),
Folate (64µg), Vitamin A (83µg),
Vitamin E (0.92mg) and Vitamin K (47µg)

MINERALS – Calcium (59mg),
Iron (2.1mg), Magnesium (28mg),
Phosphorus (35mg), Potassium (180mg),
Sodium (20mg) and Zinc (0.12mg).

[USDA national nutrient database, 2015]

Nutrient	Value per 100g
Energy	61kcal
Protein	1.5g
Fat	0.3g
Carbohydrate	14.15g
Fibre	1.8g
Sugar	3.9g

HEALTH BENEFITS

☆ **Decreased risk of birth defects**

☆ **Lowered risk of depression**

☆ **Cardiovascular benefits**

☆ **Anti-cancer**

Leeks are versatile, tasty, and easy to prepare, so don't let their relative unfamiliarity deter you. Leeks have much to offer in the way of good health and, like garlic, it's thought that much of their therapeutic effect comes from its sulfur-containing compounds, such as allicin.

Allicin is not only anti-bacterial, anti-viral and anti-fungal, but research has revealed that as allicin digests in your body, it produces sulfenic acid, a compound that neutralize dangerous free radicals faster than any other known compound.

Leeks also contain kaempferol, a natural flavonol that's also found in broccoli, kale, and cabbage. Kaempferol is impressive in its broad yet powerful potential to boost human health. Research has linked it not only to a lower risk of cancer but also a lower risk of numerous chronic diseases.

Kaempferol, and by association, leeks, is also known to protect blood vessel linings from damage, possibly by increasing production of nitric oxide (NO), which helps blood vessels to dilate and relax.

Consuming large amounts of allium vegetables, including leeks, has also been shown to reduce the risk of gastric cancer significantly as well as potentially colorectal cancer. Allium vegetables have been shown to have beneficial effects against several diseases, including cancer. Leeks have been reported to protect against stomach and colorectal cancers.

The protective effect appears to be related to the presence of organosulfur compounds and mainly allyl derivatives, which inhibit carcinogenesis in the stomach, esophagus, colon, mammary gland, and lung of experimental animals.

Leeks contain notable quantities of vitamins A and K, along with healthy amounts of folic acid, niacin, riboflavin, magnesium, and thiamin. Adequate intake of leeks during pregnancy may help prevent neural tube defects in newborns. B vitamins in leeks, in particular, may support heart health by keeping levels of homocysteine in balance (elevated levels of homocysteine are associated with heart disease, blood clots, and stroke).

Leeks also provide a concentrated source of antioxidants, even when compared to other antioxidant-rich foods.

SPICES

&

HERBS

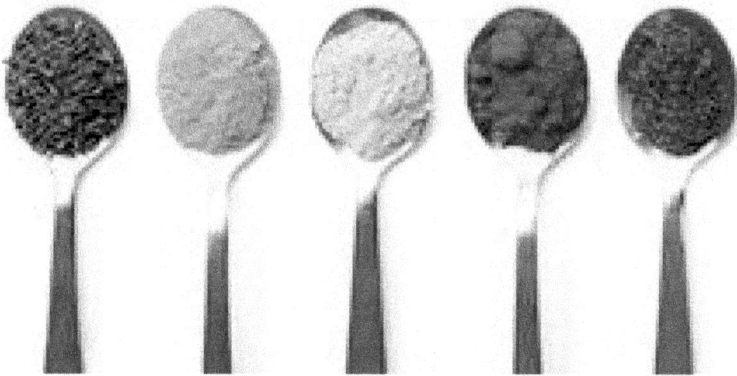

HEALTH BENEFITS OF SPICES & HERBS

Spices and herbs are mostly used for taste but they have lot of minerals, vitamins, phytonutrients (antioxidants) and essential oils. Vitamins and minerals are essential for healthy growth and immunity of the body. Phytonutrients act as antioxidants which help to eliminate free radicals from the body. Free radicals are the main causative molecules for inducing diseases like cancer, high blood pressure, diabetes and cataracts. Garlic, onion and turmeric have antiviral, antibacterial, anti-inflammatory and anticancer properties.

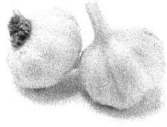

GARLIC

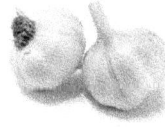

NUTRITION FACTS

VITAMINS – Vitamin C (31.2mg), Thiamin (0.2mg), Riboflavin (0.11mg), Niacin (0.7mg), Vitamin B6 (1.235mg), Folate (3µg),Vitamin E (0.08mg) and Vitamin K (1.7µg)

MINERALS – Calcium (181mg), Iron (1.7mg), Magnesium (25mg), Phosphorus (153mg), Potassium (401mg), Sodium (17mg) and Zinc (1.16mg).

[USDA national nutrient database, 2015]

Nutrient	Value per 100g
Energy	149kcal
Protein	6.36g
Fat	0.5g
Carbohydrate	33.06g
Fibre	2.1g
Sugar	1g

HEALTH BENEFITS

☆ **Anti-cancer**

☆ **Cardiovascular benefits**

☆ **Antioxidant benefits**

☆ **Essential for normal growth and development**

☆ **Reduces cholesterol**

Garlic is an underground bulb vegetable used for flavouring in cooking. It contains many phytonutrients, minerals, vitamins and antioxidants.

Allicin, is a sulphur containing compound formed during enzymatic reaction in garlic when it is cut or crushed, and contains healing effects.

Studies showed that allicin reduces cholesterol production in the liver. Allicin releases nitric acid that relaxes the blood vessels' stiffness. It blocks the platelet clot formation in blood vessels and reduces coronary artery diseases.

Allicin is found to have antiviral and antifungal qualities; it reduces the formation of cancer causing substances. Clinical studies have shown that garlic reduces the risk of cancer in the stomach, colon, pancreas and breast. Antioxidants in garlic help destroy free radicals that damage cell membranes of DNA and decrease the effects of the aging process.

Selenium in garlic, a trace element, acts as an antioxidant and reduces free radical stress.

Omega-3 fatty acids are essential for brain functions such as memory and behavioural functions; it is essential for normal growth and development. Researchers have found that it reduces the risk of diseases like cancer and heart disease.

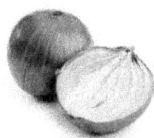

ONION

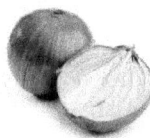

NUTRITION FACTS

VITAMINS – Vitamin C (7.4mg), Thiamin (0.046mg), Riboflavin (0.027mg), Niacin (0.116mg), Vitamin B6 (0.12mg), Folate (19μg),Vitamin E (0.02mg) and Vitamin K (0.4μg)

MINERALS – Calcium (23mg), Iron (0.21mg), Magnesium (10mg), Phosphorus (29mg), Potassium (146mg), Sodium (4mg) and Zinc (0.17mg).

[USDA national nutrient database, 2015]

Nutrient	Value per 100g
Energy	40kcal
Protein	1.1g
Fat	0.1g
Carbohydrate	9.34g
Fibre	1.7g
Sugar	4.24g

HEALTH BENEFITS

☆ **Anti-cancer**

☆ **Cardiovascular benefits**

☆ **Antioxidant benefits**

☆ **Essential for normal growth and development**

☆ **Reduces cholesterol**

☆ **Anti inflammatory**

☆ **Anti-diabetic**

Onion is an underground bulb vegetable also used as a flavouring agent in cooking. It contains lot of vitamins, minerals, and antioxidants. Phytochemical allium is converted to allicin by enzyme activity. Allicin is an antioxidant which shows anti diabetic and anti-mutagenic property.

Laboratory studies have shown that allicin reduces cholesterol production in liver cells. Allicin has anti-viral and anti-fungal activity, which helps in boosting the immune system.

Allicin releases nitric oxide that relaxes blood vessels and reduces blood pressure, coronary artery diseases, and stroke.

Chromium, a trace element in onion, helps facilitate insulin action and controls sugar levels. Quercetin, a flavonoid in onion, is anti-inflammatory, anti-diabetic, and anti-carcinogenic activity.

Manganese and selenium are trace elements which are cofactors for antioxidant enzyme Superoxide Dismutase (SOD).

Iso thiocyanate in onion helps relieve colds and phlegm. Minerals in onions are essential for metabolic activities and healthy growth.

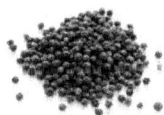

PEPPER

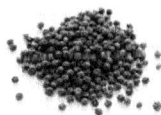

NUTRITION FACTS

VITAMINS –Thiamin (0.108mg), Riboflavin (0.18mg), Niacin (1.143mg), Vitamin B6 (0.291mg), Folate (17µg), Vitamin A (27µg), Vitamin E (1.04mg) and Vitamin K (163.7µg)

MINERALS – Calcium (443mg), Iron (9.71mg), Magnesium (171mg), Phosphorus (158mg), Potassium (1329mg), Sodium (20mg) and Zinc (1.19mg).

[USDA national nutrient database, 2015]

Nutrient	Value per 100g
Energy	251kcal
Protein	10.39g
Fat	3.26g
Carbohydrate	63.95g
Fibre	25.3g
Sugar	0.64g

HEALTH BENEFITS

☆ **Anti-cancer**

☆ **Essential for normal growth and development**

☆ **Aids indigestion**

Pepper is a dried fruit referred to as the 'king of spice.' Pepper contains an essential oil called peperine, which is an alkaloid that gives the special spicy character to pepper.

Chemicals in pepper increase the secretion of saliva and enzymes in intestine, and aid indigestion. The chemicals in pepper help to absorb vitamins and selenium.Pepper contains antioxidants such as vitamins A and C, carotene, and lutein which protect the body from diseases and cancer.

Pepper contains a good source of minerals and vitamins that are essential for a healthy body and development.

"EAT HEALTHY DAY AND NIGHT, TO KEEP YOUR FUTURE LOOKING BRIGHT"

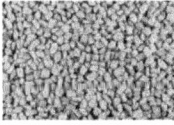

FENUGREEK

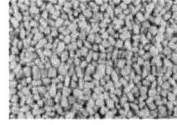

NUTRITION FACTS

VITAMINS –Vitamin C (3mg),
Thiamin (0.322mg), Riboflavin (0.366mg),
Niacin (1.64mg), Vitamin B6 (0.6mg),
Folate (57µg), Vitamin A (3µg),

MINERALS – Calcium (176mg),
Iron (33.53mg), Magnesium (191mg),
Phosphorus (296mg), Potassium (770mg),
Sodium (67mg) and Zinc (2.5mg).

[USDA national nutrient database, 2015]

Nutrient	Value per 100g
Energy	323kcal
Protein	23g
Fat	6.41g
Carbohydrate	58.35g
Fibre	24.6g

HEALTH BENEFITS

☆ Reduces colon cancer

☆ Helps sooth gastro intestinal inflammation

☆ Helps in cooling the body

☆ Reduces mucous in the sinuses

☆ Relieves constipation

☆ Aids indigestion

☆ Reduces blood cholesterol

☆ Essential for healthy growth and metabolic activity

☆ Helps cure skin problems

☆ Helps cure sore throat

☆ **Helps cure menstrual pain**

☆ **Helps control blood sugar levels**

Fenugreek is a dry seed used as spice in cooking, and contains a lot of mucilage which helps sooth gastro intestinal inflammation by coating the lining of stomach and intestine. This seed helps in cooling the body and reducing mucous in the sinuses.

Fenugreek contains soluble fibre pectin that facilitates bowel movements, relieves constipation and reduces colon cancer. It reduces blood cholesterol levels and protects the heart. The fibre in fenugreek helps in lowering the rate of glucose absorption in the intestine and controls blood sugar. These seeds can be used in a diabetic diet.

Phytochemicals in fenugreek, such as choline and yamogenin, show medicinal properties. An ammoniacal isoleucine acts on insulin secretion, and insulin controls blood sugar levels.

Vitamins and minerals found in fenugreek are essential for healthy growth and metabolic activity.

It is used in laxative, digestive, and inflammatory functions. It cures skin problems, sore throats and reduces menstrual pain. It has oestrogen-like properties and the intake of fenugreek helps to balance the mood.

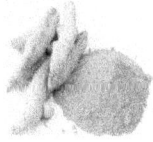

TURMERIC

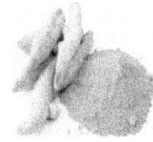

NUTRITION FACTS

VITAMINS – Vitamin C (0.7mg)
Thiamin (0.058mg), Riboflavin (0.15mg),
Niacin (1.35mg), Vitamin B6 (0.107mg),
Folate (20µg),Vitamin E (4.43mg) and
Vitamin K (13.4µg)

MINERALS – Calcium (168mg),
Iron (55mg), Magnesium (208mg),
Phosphorus (299mg), Potassium (2080mg),
Sodium (27mg) and Zinc (4.5mg).

[USDA national nutrient database, 2015]

Nutrient	Value per 100g
Energy	312kcal
Protein	9.68g
Fat	3.25g
Carbohydrate	67.14g
Fibre	22.7g
Sugar	3.21g

HEALTH BENEFITS

☆ **Anti-cancer**

☆ **Powerful antioxidant**

☆ **Anti-tumour**

☆ **Anti-ischemic**

☆ **Anti-inflammatory**

☆ **Antiviral**

☆ **Anti-bacterial**

☆ **Beneficial as a disinfectant**

☆ **Essential for normal growth and development**

☆ **Aids indigestion**

☆ **Reduces anaemia**

☆ **Reduces memory loss**

☆ **Helps prevent high blood pressure**

☆ **Helps prevent strokes**

☆ **Provides protection against infectious diseases**

Turmeric is a yellow underground stem, and is used as a spice and disinfectant in Asian countries. It contains essential oils termerone and cucumin.

Cucumin is a polytphenolic compound which acts as a powerful anti-oxidant and also has antitumor, anti-ischemic, anti-inflammatory, anti-viral, and antibacterial properties. Small amounts of turmeric per day may help reduce anaemia and memory disorders and provide protection from cancer, high blood pressure, stroke and infectious diseases.

The American Cancer Society has suggested that cucumin in turmeric inhibits the growth of tumour cells in the colon, pancreas and prostate.

Turmeric contains a good source of vitamins, fibre, and minerals that are essential for healthy growth and development.

Turmeric is a good disinfectant and is used as germ killer in Asian countries.

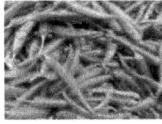

CHILI

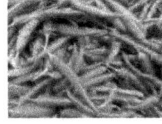

NUTRITION FACTS

VITAMINS – Vitamin C (143.7mg),
Thiamin (0.072mg), Riboflavin (0.086mg),
Niacin (1.244mg), Vitamin B6 (0.506mg),
Folate (23µg), Vitamin A (48µg),
Vitamin E (0.69mg) and Vitamin K (14µg)

MINERALS – Calcium (14mg),
Iron (1.03mg), Magnesium (23mg),
Phosphorus (43mg), Potassium (322mg),
Sodium (9mg) and Zinc (0.26mg).

[USDA national nutrient database, 2015]

Nutrient	Value per 100g
Energy	40kcal
Protein	1.87g
Fat	0.44g
Carbohydrate	8.81g
Fibre	1.5g
Sugar	5.3g

HEALTH BENEFITS

☆ **Antioxidant benefits**

☆ **Helps reduce cholesterol levels**

☆ **Helps protect the body from the effects of free radicals**

Chili is a fruit that is used fresh and dry in cooking. It contains capsaicin, an antioxidant that acts as an anti-bacterial and anti-diuretic agent. It induces the secretion of saliva and digestive juices, and also induces taste buds in the tongue.

Chili reduces cholesterol levels in the blood. It contains vitamins A and C, as well as beta-carotene and lutein which help protect the body from the effects of free radicals forming during stress and disease conditions.

"FULL OF ENERGY YOU WILL FEEL, AFTER EATING A HEALTHY MEAL"

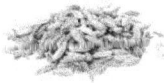

FENNEL SEEDS

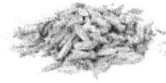

NUTRITION FACTS

VITAMINS – Vitamin C (21mg)
Thiamin (0.408mg), Riboflavin (0.353mg),
Niacin (6.05mg), Vitamin B6 (0.47mg),
Vitamin B12 (7μg), Vitamin A (135μg)

MINERALS – Calcium (1196mg),
Iron (18.54mg), Magnesium (385mg),
Phosphorus (487mg), Potassium (1694mg),
Sodium (88mg) and Zinc (3.7mg).

[USDA national nutrient database, 2015]

Nutrient	Value per 100g
Energy	345kcal
Protein	15.8g
Fat	14.87g
Carbohydrate	52.29g
Fibre	39.8g

HEALTH BENEFITS

☆ **Anti-cancer**

☆ **Antioxidant benefits**

☆ **Eliminates bad breath**

☆ **Aids digestion**

☆ **Eases constipation**

☆ **Helps lower cholesterol**

☆ **Helps increase breast milk production in nursing mothers**

☆ **Relieves colic pain in babies**

☆ **Relieves coughs and bronchitis**

☆ **Used as oil to cure joint pains**

☆ **Relieves menstrual problems in women**

☆ **Reduces obesity**

☆ **Reduces water retention**

☆ **Prevents urinary tract problems**

Fennel seeds contain numerous flavonoid antioxidants like kaempferol and quercetin. These are powerful antioxidants which act by removing harmful free radicals from the body therefore helps in protecting against cancers, infection, aging and degenerative neurological diseases.

The fibre content present in fennel seeds help ease constipation problems.

Fennel seeds also have anticancer properties as the flavonoid antioxidants along with the fibre composition help protect the colon mucus. In addition, dietary fibers bind to bile salts (produced from cholesterol) which decreases their re-absorption in the colon. This helps lower serum LDL cholesterol levels.

Fennel seeds are concentrated with minerals like copper, iron, calcium, potassium, manganese, selenium, zinc, and magnesium. They also store many vital vitamins such as vitamin A, vitamin E, vitamin C as well as many B-complex vitamins like thiamin, pyridoxine, riboflavin and niacin which are particularly concentrated in these seeds.

Fennel seeds have long been used as a remedy for indigestion and when a decoction of it is made or added as spice in food it has been found to help increase breast milk secretion in nursing mothers.

Fennel water often is used in newborn babies to relieve colic pain and help aid digestion.

Fennel seed oil is used to relieve coughs, bronchitis and as massage oil to cure joint pains.

It has been found that the antimicrobial properties of fennel seeds fight the germs that cause bad breath. Its antibacterial and anti-inflammatory properties also soothe sore gums. In addition to chewing on a fennel seeds, you can swish lukewarm fennel tea in your mouth and gargle with it to reduce bad breath.

Fennel is highly beneficial in relieving digestive problems such as indigestion, bloating, flatulence, constipation, colic, intestinal gas, heartburn, and even irritable bowel.

This herb stimulates digestion and has carminative effects that soothe the digestive tract and prevent the formation of gas. Moreover, it can help rebuild the digestive system after radiation or chemotherapy treatments.

Simply chewing a teaspoon of fennel seeds after meals aids digestion and relieves stomach pains and bloating. When suffering from indigestion, you can drink fennel tea or take one-half teaspoon of fennel seed powder along with water two times a day.

Fennel seeds help to prevent water retention and well as reducing the risk of urinary tract problems.

Consumption of fennel seeds helps suppress appetite and create a feeling of fullness which ultimately helps to reduce obesity.

Fennel seeds have also been known to relieve menstrual problems. Many factors, including stress and poor diet, can interrupt a woman's regular menstrual cycle. Consumption of fennel seeds help promote and regulate menstrual flow. The herb also has phytoestrogens that help with issues like premenstrual syndrome, menopausal disorders, and breast enlargement.

"HAVE A HEALTHY SNACK AT HAND, TO KEEP YOU FEELING GRAND"

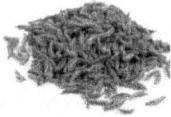

CUMIN SEEDS

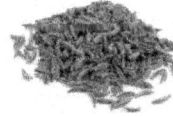

NUTRITION FACTS

VITAMINS – Vitamin C (7.7mg), Thiamin (0.628mg), Riboflavin (0.327mg), Niacin (4.579mg), Vitamin B6 (0.435mg), Folate (10μg), Vitamin A (64μg), Vitamin E (3.33mg) and Vitamin K (5.4μg)

MINERALS – Calcium (931mg), Iron (66.36mg), Magnesium (366mg), Phosphorus (499mg), Potassium (1788mg), Sodium (168mg) and Zinc (4.8mg).

[USDA national nutrient database, 2015]

Nutrient	Value per 100g
Energy	375kcal
Protein	17.81g
Fat	22.27g
Carbohydrate	44.24g
Fibre	10.5g
Sugar	2.25g

HEALTH BENEFITS

- ☆ Prevents colon cancer
- ☆ Helps with digestion
- ☆ Helps treat piles
- ☆ Helps relieve stress and anxiety
- ☆ Helps prevent respiratory disorders, asthma and bronchitis
- ☆ Helps prevent viral infections
- ☆ Beneficial for lactating mothers
- ☆ Helps with concentration and cognitive malfunction
- ☆ Prevents premature ageing
- ☆ Increases cognitive performance

☆ **Boosts immune system**

☆ **Eliminates phlegm and mucus**

☆ **Helps prevent diabetes**

☆ **Treats insect bites**

Cumin is extremely good for digestion and related problems. It helps relieve gas troubles and thereby improves digestion and appetite. Due to its essential oils, magnesium and sodium content, cumin promotes digestion and also gives relief for stomach-aches when taken with hot water.

The main cause behind piles (haemorrhoids) is constipation added with infections in the wound in the anal tract, which are also caused by constipation. Due to the high dietary fibre content as well as stimulating, antifungal and antimicrobial properties, cumin seeds act as a natural laxative in their powdered form. Adding cumin to your diet also helps in healing up of infections or wounds in the digestive and excretory system and speeds up digestion as well.

Cumin seeds have also been known to help prevent diabetes by reducing the chances of hypoglycaemia.

Cumin seeds are known as a stimulant as well as a relaxant at the same time. This property cannot be attributed to a single component alone, just as causes of insomnia cannot be attributed to a single cause. However, studies show that the proper intake of vitamins (particularly B-complex) and good digestion help to induce a sound sleep. Cumin helps in both of these factors. Some of the components of cumin essential oil are hypnotic in nature and have tranquilizing effects, which also help to relieve stress and anxiety that commonly causes insomnia.

Other health benefits of cumin seed consumption is that it helps prevent asthma, bronchitis and prevents respiratory disorders. The cumin seeds help by loosening up the accumulated phlegm and mucus in the respiratory tracts and makes it easier to eliminate them from the system via sneezing or coughing up and spitting. By eliminating as much of the mucus and phlegm as possible, it can inhibit the formation of additional material and help to heal the initial condition that led to its formation in the first place.

The common cold is a viral infection which affects our body frequently when our immune system becomes weakened or vulnerable. Again, the essential oils present in cumin act as disinfectants and help fight viral infections which can cause the common cold. Cumin also suppresses the development of coughing in the respiratory system since it dries up the excess mucus. Cumin is rich in iron and has considerable amount of vitamin C, which are essential for a healthy immune system and keeps infections from forming or becoming worse. Vitamin C is also a antioxidant, so it defends against other infections and toxins as well, further boosting the immune system.

The rich source of iron in cumin is thus very good for lactating mothers as well as for women who are undergoing menses or who are pregnant, since they are more in need of iron than others. Moreover, cumin is said to help ease and increase secretion of milk in lactating women due to the presence of thymol, which tends to increase secretions from our glands, including milk, which is a secretion from the mammary glands.

The amount of iron in cumin leads to increased haemoglobin production and subsequent prevention of anaemia, but that increased blood flow has other benefits as well. When your blood circulation is in top form, adequate amounts of oxygen are able to reach the organs and the brain, leading to optimal performance of those bodily systems. Proper amounts of oxygen and iron in the brain lead to increased cognitive performance and a decrease in cognitive disorders like Alzheimer's disease and dementia. For other organs, increased oxygenation increases efficiency and speeds up the metabolism, which can boost your overall health, increase strength, and prevent signs of aging.

Vitamin E present in cumin seeds is good for the maintenance of skin and the prevention of premature aging symptoms. It keeps the skin young and glowing.

Cumin seeds have detoxifying and chemo preventive properties, and accelerates the secretion of detoxifying and anti-carcinogenic enzymes from the glands, as it also does to other secretions. Furthermore, it has beneficial antioxidants like vitamin C and vitamin A within its chemical makeup, in addition to those essential oils.. The antioxidants found in cumin are particularly good for colon cancer prevention.

Cumin is also beneficial in treating insect bites and painful stings.

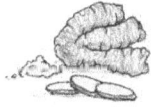

GINGER

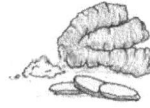

NUTRITION FACTS

VITAMINS – Vitamin C (0.7mg), Thiamin (0.046mg), Riboflavin (0.17mg), Niacin (9.62mg), Vitamin B6 (0.626mg), Folate (13µg), Vitamin A (2µg), and Vitamin K (0.8µg)

MINERALS – Calcium (114mg), Iron (19.8mg), Magnesium (214mg), Phosphorus (168mg), Potassium (1320mg), Sodium (27mg) and Zinc (3.64mg).

[USDA national nutrient database, 2015]

Nutrient	Value per 100g
Energy	335kcal
Protein	8.98g
Fat	4.24g
Carbohydrate	71.62g
Fibre	14.1g
Sugar	3.39g

HEALTH BENEFITS

☆ **Helps with digestion**

☆ **Helps to relieve gastrointestinal irritation**

☆ **Prevents nausea**

☆ **Reduces pain**

☆ **Anti-inflammatory**

Ginger is known to help relieve gastrointestinal irritation, stimulate saliva and bile production and suppress gastric contractions and movement of food and fluids through the gastrointestinal tract.

Chewing raw ginger or drinking ginger tea is a common home remedy for nausea. This is particularly useful for pregnant women who experience morning sickness as they can safely consume ginger to relieve nausea and vomiting, often in the form of ginger lozenges or candies.

Research has shown that daily consumption of ginger has helped reduce exercise-induced muscle pain by 25%.

Ginger has also been found to reduce the symptoms of dysmenorrhoea (severe pain during a menstrual cycle).

Consumption of ginger has also been known to help treat inflammation especially associated with osteoarthritis.

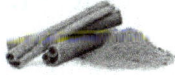

CINAMMON

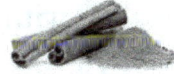

NUTRITION FACTS

VITAMINS – Vitamin C (3.8mg), Thiamin (0.022mg), Riboflavin (0.041mg), Niacin (1.332mg), Vitamin B6 (0.158mg), Folate (6µg), Vitamin A (15µg), Vitamin E (2.32mg) and Vitamin K (31.2µg)

MINERALS – Calcium (1002mg), Iron (8.32mg), Magnesium (60mg), Phosphorus (64mg), Potassium (431mg), Sodium (10mg) and Zinc (1.83mg).

[USDA national nutrient database, 2015]

Nutrient	Value per 100g
Energy	247kcal
Protein	3.99g
Fat	1.24g
Carbohydrate	80.59g
Fibre	53.1g
Sugar	2.17g

HEALTH BENEFITS

☆ **Antioxidant benefits**

☆ **Anti-inflammatory properties**

☆ **Cut the risk of heart disease**

☆ **Beneficial for type 2 diabetics**

☆ **Reduces levels of total cholesterol**

☆ **Beneficial effects on neurodegenerative diseases**

☆ **Protective against cancer**

☆ **Helps fight bacterial and fungal infections**

☆ **Helps prevent tooth decay and reduce bad breath**

☆ **May help fight the HIV virus**

Cinnamon is loaded with antioxidants which help protect the body from oxidative damage caused by free radicals.

Cinnamon also has anti-inflammatory properties as it helps the body fight infections and repair tissue damage.

Cinnamon has been linked with reduced risk of heart disease, the world's most common cause of premature death.

Consumption of cinnamon on a daily basis is very beneficial for people with type 2 diabetes. Cinnamon can help improve sensitivity to the hormone insulin. Insulin is known to be one of the key hormones that regulate metabolism and energy use. It is also essential for the transport of blood sugar from the bloodstream and into cells. Thus it lowers blood sugar levels and has a powerful anti-diabetic effect.

It has also been shown to reduces levels of total cholesterol, LDL cholesterol and triglycerides, while HDL cholesterol remains stable

Cinnamon may also have beneficial effects on neurodegenerative diseases. Neurodegenerative diseases are characterized by progressive loss of the structure or function of brain cells.

Alzheimer's disease and Parkinson's disease are two of the most common types.

Two compounds found in cinnamon appear to inhibit the build up of a protein called tau in the brain, which is one of the hallmarks of Alzheimer's disease .

Cinnamon have been shown to have possible effects on preventing cancer. It acts by reducing the growth of cancer cells and the formation of blood vessels in tumours, and appears to be toxic to cancer cells, causing cell death.

Cinnamaldehyde, the main active component of cinnamon, may help fight various kinds of infection.

Cinnamon oil has been shown to effectively treat respiratory tract infections caused by fungi.

It can also inhibit the growth of certain bacteria, including Listeria and Salmonella.

The antimicrobial effects of cinnamon may also help prevent tooth decay and reduce bad breath .

HIV is a virus that slowly breaks down the immune system, which can eventually lead to AIDS if untreated. Cinnamon extracted from Cassia varieties is thought to help fight against HIV-1. This is the most common strain of the HIV virus in humans. Human trials are needed to confirm these effects.

"TO KEEP YOUR HEALTH ON TRACK, FRUITS AND VEGGIES YOU SHOULDN'T LACK"

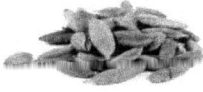

CARDAMOM

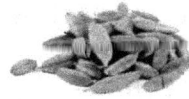

NUTRITION FACTS

VITAMINS – Vitamin C (21mg), Thiamin (0.198mg), Riboflavin (0.182mg), Niacin (1.102mg) and Vitamin B6 (0.23mg),

MINERALS – Calcium (383mg), Iron (13.97mg), Magnesium (229mg), Phosphorus (178mg), Potassium (1119mg), Sodium (18mg) and Zinc (7.47mg).

[USDA national nutrient database, 2015]

Nutrient	Value per 100g
Energy	311kcal
Protein	10.76g
Fat	6.7g
Carbohydrate	68.47g
Fibre	28g

HEALTH BENEFITS

☆ **Aids in digestion**

☆ **Helps body eliminate waste through the kidneys**

☆ **Good detoxifier**

☆ **Antidepressant**

☆ **Eradicates bad breath**

☆ **Oral health**

☆ **Relieve cold and flu symptoms**

☆ **Anti-cancer**

☆ **Lowers blood pressure**

☆ **Prevents blood clots**

☆ **Antioxidant benefits**

☆ **Anti-inflammatory benefits**

☆ **Helps get rid of hiccups**

Cardamom is related to ginger and can be used in a similar way to counteract digestive problems. It can be used to combat nausea, acidity, bloating, gas, heartburn, loss of appetite, constipation, and much more.

Cardamom is also a spice which is known to help the body eliminate waste through the kidneys. Cardamom is such a good detoxifier due to its diuretic properties. It helps clean out the urinary tract, bladder, and kidneys, removing waste, salt, excess water, toxins, and combating infections too.

By chewing on cardamom it will help eradicate bad breath. Apart from helping with bad breath, cardamom is used for mouth ulcers and infections of the mouth and throat.

Yet to be proven but Ayurvedic medicine swears by the tea as a means to fight depression thus cardamom acts as a good antidepressant.

This spice has been known to be used to help prevent and relieve cold and flu symptoms. It's also used for bronchitis and coughs.

Research on animals have shown that cardamom protects against, inhibits growth, and even kills some cancers.

Due to cardamom being rich in fibre it has known to significantly lower blood pressure and prevent dangerous blood clots by preventing platelet aggregation and the sticking to the artery walls.

Many of the vitamins, phytonutrients, and essential oils in cardamom act as antioxidants, cleaning up free radicals and resisting cellular aging.

It inhibits the growth of viruses, bacteria, fungus, and mold by the volatile essential oils present within the spice.

Cardamom has similar properties to ginger and turmeric as they consist of anti-inflammatory properties that limit pain and swelling, especially in mucus membranes, the mouth, and throat.

Finally cardamom is also an anti-spasmodic that can help get rid of hiccups. This also applies to other involuntary muscle spasms, like stomach and intestinal cramps.

"TO LOOK THE BEST, EAT THE BEST"

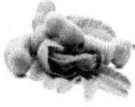

TAMARIND

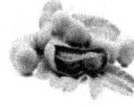

NUTRITION FACTS

VITAMINS – Vitamin C (3.5mg), Thiamin (0.428mg), Riboflavin (0.152mg), Niacin (1.938mg), Vitamin B6 (0.066mg), Folate (14µg), Vitamin A (2µg), Vitamin E (0.1mg) and Vitamin K (2.8µg)

MINERALS – Calcium (74mg), Iron (2.8mg), Magnesium (92mg), Phosphorus (113mg), Potassium 628mg), Sodium (28mg) and Zinc (0.1mg).

[USDA national nutrient database, 2015]

Nutrient	Value per 100g
Energy	239kcal
Protein	2.8g
Fat	0.6g
Carbohydrate	62.5g
Fibre	5.1g
Sugar	38.8g

HEALTH BENEFITS

☆ **Antioxidant benefits**

☆ **Helps gastric and digestive problems**

☆ **Helps improve bowel movement**

☆ **Useful to treat bilious disorders**

☆ **Reduces malaria fever**

☆ **Protection from vitamin C deficiency**

☆ **Helps treat piles**

☆ **Anti-cancer**

☆ **Helps lower cholesterol**

☆ **Helps treat sore throats**

☆ **Useful in treating jaundice and ulcers**

☆ **Antioxidant benefits**

Tamarind has multiple benefits. Tamarind is used as an Ayurvedic medicine for gastric problem and digestion problems.

The pulp which comes from the pods of the tamarind tree is known to be used as a mild laxative that improves general sluggishness of the bowels. Thus can help improve bowel movements.

Tamarind leaves are used in herbal tea for reducing malaria fever and is very useful in treating bilious disorders. Being acidic it excites the bile and other juices in the body.

The spice helps lower cholesterol level in the body and thus benefits the cardiovascular system.

Sore throat is treated when gargled with dilute tamarind pulp.

Decoction of tamarind leaves is useful in treating jaundice and ulcers.

It has also been known that dilute tamarind decoction can help in destroying the stomach worms in children.

Other benefits of consuming tamarind include its protection from Vitamin C deficiency, helps heal the inflammation of the skin and is a good source of antioxidants that helps fight against cancer as well as being used as a blood purifier

Tamarind seeds are used in preparations of eye drops that treat dry eye syndrome and the juice extracted from tamarind flowers are used for treating piles.

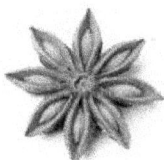

CLOVES

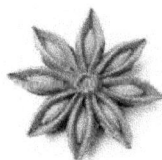

NUTRITION FACTS

VITAMINS – Vitamin C (0.2mg), Thiamin (0.158mg), Riboflavin (0.22mg), Niacin (1.56mg), Vitamin B6 (0.391mg), Folate (25μg), Vitamin A (8μg), Vitamin E (8.82mg) and Vitamin K (141.8μg)

MINERALS – Calcium (632mg), Iron (11.83mg), Magnesium (259mg), Phosphorus (104mg), Potassium (1020mg), Sodium (277mg) and Zinc (2.32mg).

[USDA national nutrient database, 2015]

Nutrient	Value per 100g
Energy	274kcal
Protein	5.97g
Fat	13g
Carbohydrate	65.53g
Fibre	33.9g
Sugar	2.38g

HEALTH BENEFITS

☆ **Provides relief from headaches**

☆ **Boosts immune system**

☆ **Aids in digestion**

☆ **Protects liver against infection**

☆ **Effective against bacterial infection**

☆ **Beneficial in preserving bone density**

☆ **Helps in controlling blood sugar levels**

☆ **Provides relief from inflammation and pain**

☆ **Anti-cancer**

☆ **Aids in treating gum disease**

Cloves help to improve digestion by stimulating the secretion of digestive enzymes. Cloves can be roasted, powdered, and taken with honey for relief in digestive disorders.

Cloves have been tested for their antibacterial properties against a number of human pathogens. The extracts of cloves help fight against bacteria thus are known for their antibacterial properties.

The high amounts of antioxidants present in cloves, are ideal for protecting the organs from the effects of free radicals, especially the liver.

Research have shown that cloves have anti-carcinogenic properties and have been helpful in controlling lung cancer in their early stages.

Studies have shown that extracts from cloves imitate insulin in certain ways and help in controlling blood sugar levels. Thus helping to control diabetes.

The hydro-alcoholic extracts of cloves help preserve bone density and the mineral content of bone, as well as increasing tensile strength of bones in cases of osteoporosis. The hydro-alcoholic compounds include phenolic compounds such as eugenol and its derivatives, such as flavones, isoflavones and flavonoids.

Cloves are effective in developing and protecting the immune system. The compounds present in the dried flower bud of the clove helps in improving the immune system by increasing the white blood cell count, thereby improving delayed type hypersensitivity.

Studies have shown that cloves have been known to reduce inflammation caused by oedema.

Gum diseases such as gingivitis and periodontitis have also been known to be treated by cloves. Cloves can also be used for toothaches due to their pain-killing properties.

Cloves can help cure headachesby making a paste of a few cloves and mixing it with a dash of rock salt which is then added to a glass of milk. This mixture reduces headaches quickly and effectively.

"TO PREVENT FUTURE DISMAY, START HEALTHY EATING TODAY"

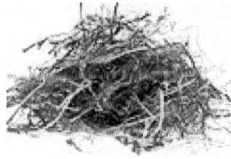

SAFFRON

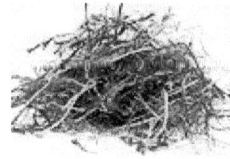

NUTRITION FACTS

VITAMINS – Vitamin C (80.8mg),
Thiamin (0.115mg), Riboflavin (0.267mg),
Niacin (1.46mg), Vitamin B6 (1.01mg),
Folate (93µg), and Vitamin A (27µg),

MINERALS – Calcium (111mg),
Iron (11.1mg), Magnesium (264mg),
Phosphorus (252mg), Potassium (1724mg),
Sodium (148mg) and Zinc (1.09mg).

[USDA national nutrient database, 2015]

Nutrient	Value per 100g
Energy	310kcal
Protein	11.43g
Fat	5.85g
Carbohydrate	65.37g
Fibre	3.9g

HEALTH BENEFITS

☆ **Helps prevent diseases**

☆ **Antioxidant benefits**

☆ **Therapeutic applications**

☆ **Anti-depressant**

☆ **Favours cell formation and repair**

☆ **Maintains blood pressure**

☆ **Prevents heart problems**

☆ **Skin benefits**

☆ **Treatment of acne and blemishes**

Saffron is mostly known for its inclusion in food items. However it has very significant nutrients and chemical compounds which are beneficial in providing medicinal benefits.

The main benefit of saffron is that it consists of many plant derived chemical components which are known to help prevent diseases thus promoting a healthier body.

Saffron consists of components like carotenoid that are antioxidants which are beneficial to the body. These prevent free radical reactions which produce harmful by-compounds and diseases.

Saffron is also used in various types of therapies such as body healing, detoxification and also in the spas.

The active components in the saffron make our body lose its depressing characteristics making it a good anti-depressant.

Potassium, found in saffron, is a necessary source that favours cell formation and repair as well as helping to maintain blood pressure and prevent heart problems.

Saffron consists of very useful components such as iron, needed to form haemoglobin, as well as calcium, vitamins, proteins which help maintain optimum health.

Saffron benefits the skin in several ways as it has natural skin lightening qualities as well as making the skin more radiant.

The antifungal content of saffron also makes it an effective component for the treatment of acne, blemishes and blackheads.

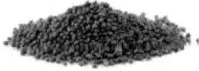

MUSTARD SEEDS

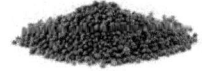

NUTRITION FACTS

VITAMINS – Vitamin C (7.1mg), Thiamin (0.805mg), Riboflavin (0.261mg), Niacin (4.733mg), Vitamin B6 (0.397mg), Folate (162µg), Vitamin A (2µg), Vitamin E (5.07mg) and Vitamin K (5.4µg)

MINERALS – Calcium (266mg), Iron (9.21mg), Magnesium (370mg), Phosphorus (828mg), Potassium (738mg), Sodium (13mg) and Zinc (6.08mg).

[USDA national nutrient database, 2015]

Nutrient	Value per 100g
Energy	508kcal
Protein	26.08g
Fat	36.24g
Carbohydrate	28.09g
Fibre	12.2g
Sugar	6.79g

HEALTH BENEFITS

☆ **Anti-cancer**

☆ **Source of relief for rheumatoid arthritis**

☆ **Reduces migraines**

☆ **Assist treating blood pressure and menopausal relief**

☆ **Anti-asthma**

☆ **Hydrates the skin and slows aging**

☆ **Fights infections**

☆ **Great nutrient for faster growing and stronger hair**

☆ **Removes odour**

☆ **Relieves muscle pain**

☆ Treats cold, flu and back pains

Mustard seeds help to inhibit the growth of cancer cells and also act as an antioxidant. Due to the presence of compounds like glucosinolates and mirosinase.

Relief from rheumatic arthritis can occur when mustard seeds are consumed, The selenium and magnesium content in the seeds help in providing relief from this problem.

Migraine occurrence also reduces owing to the magnesium content present in the mustard seed.

Mustard seeds are known to get rid of flu like symptoms and back pain.

Mustard seeds are a good source of dietary fibres that improve digestion in the body. Thus making the bowel movements better.

Mustard seeds are comprised of copper, iron, magnesium and selenium which assist in the treatment of blood pressure and menopause relief as well as prevention of asthma attacks.

Mustard seeds hydrate the skin by removing the impurities and thus

Fight off infections is another key benefit of mustard seed consumption in our daily food.

Increase in hair growth and strength when consuming mustard seeds are due to the vitamin A content as it's a great nutrient for hair growth. It also conditions the hair to give it a good shine and bounce.

Other uses are that it removes odour, relieves muscle pain, relieves congestion caused by bad cough or cold, relieves spasms and back pains. Finally it can also be used to lower fever as it helps release toxins from the body.

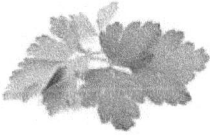

CORIANDER

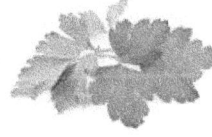

NUTRITION FACTS

VITAMINS – Vitamin C (566.7mg),
Thiamin (1.252mg), Riboflavin (1.5mg),
Niacin (10.707mg), Vitamin B6 (0.61mg),
Folate (274µg), Vitamin A (293µg),
Vitamin E (1.03mg) and
Vitamin K (1359.5µg)

MINERALS – Calcium (1246mg),
Iron (42.46mg), Magnesium (694mg),
Phosphorus (481mg), Potassium (4466mg),
Sodium (211mg) and Zinc (4.72mg).

[USDA national nutrient database, 2015]

Nutrient	Value per 100g
Energy	279kcal
Protein	21.93g
Fat	4.78g
Carbohydrate	52.1g
Fibre	10.4g
Sugar	7.27g

HEALTH BENEFITS

☆ **Clears up skin disorders such as eczema, dryness and fungal infections**

☆ **Helps reduce swelling due to kidney malfunction or anaemia**

☆ **Prevents nausea, vomiting and stomach disorders**

☆ **Clears ulcers and freshens breath**

☆ **Cures diarrhoea and stimulates digestion**

☆ **Protects eyes from conjunctivitis**

☆ **Prevents and cures smallpox**

☆ **Reduces blood pressure**

☆ **Keeps bones healthy**

Coriander consists of both essential oils and linoleic acid which possess anti-rheumatic and anti-arthritic properties. They help to reduce the swelling that is caused by these two conditions. Thus reducing skin inflammation. The antioxidant properties of coriander help clear up skin disorders such as eczema, dryness and fungal infections.

The acids present in coriander, like linoleic acid, oleic acid, palmitic acid, stearic acid and ascorbic acid (vitamin C) help reduce cholesterol levels in the body.

The essential oils such as Borneol and Linalool found in coriander aid in digestion, proper functioning of the liver and bonding of bowels, while also helping to reduce diarrhoea.

Coriander also helps prevent nausea, vomiting, and other stomach disorders.

Consumption of coriander has been shown to significantly reduce blood pressure in patients suffering from hypertension.

Citronelol, a component of essential oils in coriander, is an excellent antiseptic. Additionally, other components have antimicrobial and healing effects which keep wounds and ulcers in the mouth from worsening. They help speed up the healing process of ulcers and also freshen breath.

The high iron content in coriander help people who suffer from anaemia.

Coriander has a good source of calcium which is great for healthy bones. It also aids digestion and cures diarrhoea.

The essential oils in coriander are rich in antimicrobial, antioxidant, anti-infectious and detoxifying components and acids. The presence of vitamin C and iron strengthens the immune system as well. These properties help prevent and cure smallpox, and they can also reduce the pain and have a soothing effect on smallpox patients.

Coriander is a natural stimulant, and it regulates proper secretion from the endocrine glands, and that hormonal impact means that it helps regulate proper menstrual cycles and reduces the associated pain during a woman's period.

Coriander is loaded with antioxidants, vitamin A, vitamin C and minerals like phosphorous in its essential oils, which prevents vision disorders, macular degeneration and it reduces strain and stress on the eyes. It also consists of beta-carotene in the leaves, which prevent a number of other diseases that affect the eye, and can even reverse the effects of vision degradation in aging patients. It is a very good disinfectant and has antimicrobial properties that protect the eyes from contagious diseases like conjunctivitis.

Consumption of coriander helps increase the secretion of insulin from the pancreas which subsequently increases the insulin level in the blood. This regulates absorption of sugar and thus results in the drop in sugar level in the blood. Thus it is beneficial for diabetic patients in order to lower their chances of dangerous spikes and drops in their blood sugar levels, and to ensure other normal metabolic functions as well.

Other benefits of coriander include helping to cure inflammation, spasms and ulcers.

"WHEN EATING HEALTHY YOU CAN'T GO WRONG IN KEEPING YOUR BODY LEAN AND STRONG"

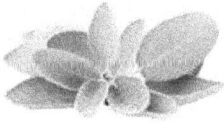

SAGE

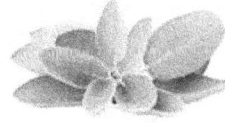

NUTRITION FACTS

VITAMINS – Vitamin C (32.4mg),
Thiamin (0.754mg), Riboflavin (0.336mg),
Niacin (5.72mg), Vitamin B6 (2.69mg),
Folate (274µg), Vitamin A (295µg),
Vitamin E (7.48mg) and
Vitamin K (1714.5µg)

MINERALS – Calcium (1652mg),
Iron (28.12mg), Magnesium (428mg),
Phosphorus (91mg), Potassium (1070mg),
Sodium (11mg) and Zinc (4.7mg).

[USDA national nutrient database, 2015]

Nutrient	Value per 100g
Energy	315kcal
Protein	10.63g
Fat	12.78g
Carbohydrate	60.73g
Fibre	40.3g
Sugar	1.71g

HEALTH BENEFITS

☆ **Antioxidant benefits**

☆ **Helps lower blood glucose and cholesterol**

☆ **Anti-inflammatory, antifungal and antimicrobial effects**

Sage has high antioxidant benefits which help protect the body's cells from damage caused by free radicals. This often results in cell death, impaired immunity, and chronic disease.

Studies have shown that sage is known to help lower blood glucose and cholesterol.

As per many spices and herbs, sage is also known to have anti-inflammatory, antifungal and antimicrobial effects.

"TO STAY LOOKING FINE, MAKE HEALTHY CHOICES WHEN YOU DINE"

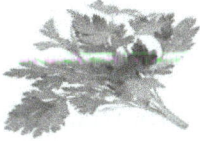

PARSLEY

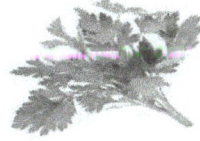

NUTRITION FACTS

VITAMINS – Vitamin C (125mg), Thiamin (0.196mg), Riboflavin (2.383mg), Niacin (9.943mg), Vitamin B6 (0.9mg), Folate (180µg), Vitamin A (97µg), Vitamin E (8.96mg) and Vitamin K (1359.5µg)

MINERALS – Calcium (1140mg), Iron (22.04mg), Magnesium (400mg), Phosphorus (436mg), Potassium (2683mg), Sodium (452mg) and Zinc (5.44mg).

[USDA national nutrient database, 2015]

Nutrient	Value per 100g
Energy	292kcal
Protein	26.63g
Fat	5.48g
Carbohydrate	50.64g
Fibre	26.7g
Sugar	7.27g

HEALTH BENEFITS

☆ **Anti-cancer**

☆ **Helps decrease tumour size**

☆ **Helps prevent diabetes**

☆ **Improves bone health**

Parsley contains a high concentration of the flavanol myricetin which has been shown to have chemo preventive effects on skin cancer.

Recent studies have shown that apigenin found in parsley has been known to decrease tumour size in an aggressive form of breast cancer. Researchers say that this shows a promising non-toxic treatment for cancer in the future.

The flavanol myricetin has shown to help lower blood sugars as well as decrease insulin resistance and provide anti-inflammatory and anti-hyperlipidemia effects.

Parsley consists of adequate amounts of potassium which helps improve bone health by acting as a modifier of bone matrix proteins thus improving calcium absorption and reducing urinary excretion of calcium.

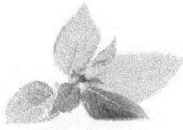

BASIL

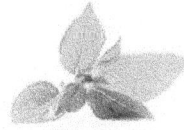

NUTRITION FACTS

VITAMINS – Vitamin C (0.8mg), Thiamin (0.08mg), Riboflavin (1.2mg), Niacin (4.9mg), Vitamin B6 (1.34mg), Folate (310µg), Vitamin A (37µg), Vitamin E (10.7mg) and Vitamin K (1714.5µg)

MINERALS – Calcium (2240mg), Iron (89.8mg), Magnesium (711mg), Phosphorus (274mg), Potassium (2630mg), Sodium (76mg) and Zinc (7.1mg).

[USDA national nutrient database, 2015]

Nutrient	Value per 100g
Energy	233kcal
Protein	22.98g
Fat	4.07g
Carbohydrate	47.75g
Fibre	37.7g
Sugar	1.71g

HEALTH BENEFITS

☆ **Anti-bacterial properties**

☆ **Helps decrease tumour size**

☆ **Cardiovascular benefits**

☆ **Anti-inflammatory effects**

Basil has been shown to provide protection against unwanted bacterial growth.

Basil improves cardiovascular health due to containing a good source of magnesium by prompting muscles and blood vessels to relax, thus improving blood flow and therefore lessening the risk of irregular heart rhythms.

Basil is classified as an anti-inflammatory food due to the enzyme-inhibiting effect of the eugenol present in basil that can provide important healing benefits along with symptomatic relief for individuals with inflammatory health problems like rheumatoid arthritis or inflammatory bowel conditions.

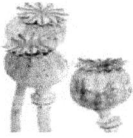

POPPY SEED

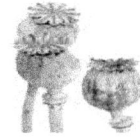

NUTRITION FACTS

VITAMINS – Vitamin C (1mg),
Thiamin (0.854mg), Riboflavin (0.1mg),
Niacin (0.896mg), Vitamin B6 (0.247mg),
Folate (82µg) and Vitamin E (1.77mg)

MINERALS – Calcium (1438mg),
Iron (9.76mg), Magnesium (347mg),
Phosphorus (870mg), Potassium (719mg),
Sodium (26mg) and Zinc (7.9mg).

[USDA national nutrient database, 2015]

Nutrient	Value per 100g
Energy	525kcal
Protein	17.99g
Fat	41.56g
Carbohydrate	28.13g
Fibre	19.5g
Sugar	2.99g

HEALTH BENEFITS

☆ **Anti-cancer**

☆ **Prevents constipation and helps digestion**

☆ **Cardiovascular benefits**

☆ **Helps lower cholesterol**

☆ **Prevents osteoporosis**

☆ **Fights against bacteria**

☆ **Helps prevent insomnia**

☆ **Prevents kidney stone formation**

☆ **Eases skin inflammations**

Poppy seeds contain oleic acid which inhibits the activity levels of the gene that triggers breast cancer.

Poppy seeds are a rich source of fibre which helps with digestion and thus prevents or eases constipation. The dietary fibre found in poppy seeds also aids to lower cholesterol.

Due to the high content of fatty acids in poppy seeds help prevent coronary artery disease and might help reduce your risk of having a stroke.

Poppy seeds are an excellent source of calcium and phosphorus which can help keep the bones strong and help prevent the development of osteoporosis.

Poppy seeds consumption helps boost the immune system due to the rich content of iron and zinc. Zinc helps stimulates the body's production of bacteria fighting cells whilst iron oxygenates the blood.

Natural supply of alkaloids present in poppy seeds are extremely helpful for treating nervous disorders.

Poppy seeds also have a naturally relaxing effect which can help with having a regular sleeping pattern and thus preventing insomnia.

Poppy seeds also significantly reduce the risk of heart attacks and the rich source of iron helps keep up your bodies energy level.

Kidney stone formation can also be prevented as poppy seeds contain oxalates that can help reduce your body's absorption of calcium.

Finally due to the high content of linoleum acid poppy seeds can be used as a natural remedy for eczema and can also ease skin inflammations.

INDEX

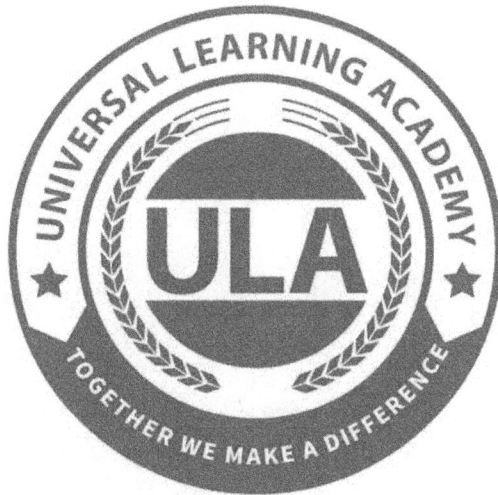